T0259422

Management of Brain Metastases

Guest Editors

ANTHONY L. D'AMBROSIO, MD
GANESH RAO, MD

NEUROSURGERY
CLINICS OF NORTH AMERICA

www.neurosurgery.theclinics.com

Consulting Editors

ANDREW T. PARSA, MD, PhD
PAUL C. McCORMICK, MD, MPH

January 2011 • Volume 22 • Number 1

SAUNDERS an imprint of ELSEVIER, Inc.

W.B. SAUNDERS COMPANY
A Division of Elsevier Inc.

1600 John F. Kennedy Blvd. • Suite 1800 • Philadelphia, PA 19103-2899

http://www.theclinics.com

NEUROSURGERY CLINICS OF NORTH AMERICA Volume 22, Number 1
January 2011 ISSN 1042-3680, ISBN-13: 978-1-4557-0471-2

Editor: Ruth Malwitz
Developmental Editor: Donald Mumford

© 2011 Elsevier Inc. All rights reserved.

This journal and the individual contributions contained in it are protected under copyright by Elsevier, and the following terms and conditions apply to their use:

Photocopying

Single photocopies of single articles may be made for personal use as allowed by national copyright laws. Permission of the Publisher and payment of a fee is required for all other photocopying, including multiple or systematic copying, copying for advertising or promotional purposes, resale, and all forms of document delivery. Special rates are available for educational institutions that wish to make photocopies for non-profit educational classroom use. For information on how to seek permission visit www.elsevier.com/permissions or call: (+44) 1865 843830 (UK)/(+1) 215 239 3804 (USA).

Derivative Works

Subscribers may reproduce tables of contents or prepare lists of articles including abstracts for internal circulation within their institutions. Permission of the Publisher is required for resale or distribution outside the institution. Permission of the Publisher is required for all other derivative works, including compilations and translations (please consult www.elsevier.com/permissions).

Electronic Storage or Usage

Permission of the Publisher is required to store or use electronically any material contained in this journal, including any article or part of an article (please consult www.elsevier.com/permissions). Except as outlined above, no part of this publication may be reproduced, stored in a retrieval system or transmitted in any form or by any means, electronic, mechanical, photocopying, recording or otherwise, without prior written permission of the Publisher.

Notice

No responsibility is assumed by the Publisher for any injury and/or damage to persons or property as a matter of products liability, negligence or otherwise, or from any use or operation of any methods, products, instructions or ideas contained in the material herein. Because of rapid advances in the medical sciences, in particular, independent verification of diagnoses and drug dosages should be made.

Although all advertising material is expected to conform to ethical (medical) standards, inclusion in this publication does not constitute a guarantee or endorsement of the quality or value of such product or of the claims made of it by its manufacturer.

Neurosurgery Clinics of North America (ISSN 1042-3680) is published quarterly by Elsevier Inc., 360 Park Avenue South, New York, NY 10010-1710. Months of issue are January, April, July, and October. Business and Editorial Offices: 1600 John F. Kennedy Blvd., Suite 1800, Philadelphia, PA 19103-2899. Customer Service Office: 11830 Westline Industrial Drive, St. Louis, MO 63146. Periodicals postage paid at New York, NY, and additional mailing offices. Subscription prices are $317.00 per year (US individuals), $492.00 per year (US institutions), $347.00 per year (Canadian individuals), $601.00 per year (Canadian institutions), $443.00 per year (international individuals), $601.00 per year (international institutions), $156.00 per year (US students), and $214.00 per year (international students). International air speed delivery is included in all *Clinics* subscription prices. All prices are subject to change without notice. **POSTMASTER:** Send address changes to *Neurosurgery Clinics of North America*, Elsevier Periodicals Customer Service, 11830 Westline Industrial Drive, St. Louis, MO 63146. **Customer Service: 1-800-654-2452 (US and Canada). From outside the US and Canada, call: 1-314-453-7041. Fax: 1-314-453-5170. E-mail: JournalsCustomerService-usa@elsevier.com (for print support) and journalsonlinesupport-usa@elsevier.com (for online support).**

Reprints. For copies of 100 or more, of articles in this publication, please contact the Commercial Reprints Department, Elsevier Inc., 360 Park Avenue South, New York, NY 10010-1710. Tel. (212) 633-3812; Fax: (212) 462-1935; E-mail: reprints@elsevier.com.

Neurosurgery Clinics of North America is covered in *MEDLINE/PubMed (Index Medicus), EMBASE/Excerpta Medica, and Current Contents/Clinical Medicine (CC/CM)*.

Printed in the United States of America.

Cover image copyright © 2010, The Johns Hopkins University. All rights reserved. Courtesy of Ian Suk, Johns Hopkins University; with permission.

Printed and bound by CPI Group (UK) Ltd, Croydon, CR0 4YY

Transferred to Digital Print 2011

Contributors

CONSULTING EDITORS

ANDREW T. PARSA, MD, PhD
Associate Professor; Principal Investigator,
Brain Tumor Research Center; Reza and
Georgianna Khatib Endowed Chair in Skull
Base Tumor Surgery, Department of
Neurological Surgery, University of California,
San Francisco, San Francisco, California

PAUL C. MCCORMICK, MD, MPH, FACS
Herbert & Linda Gallen Professor of
Neurological Surgery, Department of
Neurological Surgery, Columbia University
Medical Center, New York, New York

GUEST EDITORS

ANTHONY L. D'AMBROSIO, MD
Assistant Professor of Neurological Surgery,
Department of Neurological Surgery,
Columbia University College of Physicians
and Surgeons, New York, New York; Director
of Neuro-Oncology, Blumenthal Cancer
Center, The Valley Hospital, Ridgewood; Chief,
Division of Neurological Surgery, St Joseph's
Regional Medical Center, Paterson,
New Jersey

GANESH RAO, MD
Assistant Professor, Department of
Neurosurgery, The University of Texas,
MD Anderson Cancer Center,
Houston, Texas

AUTHORS

MUHAMMAD M. ABD-EL-BARR, MD, PhD
Department of Neurosurgery, University of
Florida, Gainesville, Florida

DAVID W. ANDREWS, MD
Professor of Neurosurgery, Department of
Neurosurgery, Thomas Jefferson University,
Philadelphia, Pennsylvania

KARA D. BEASLEY, DO, MBe
Doctor of Osteopathic Medicine, Geisinger
Medical Center, Danville; Philadelphia College
of Osteopathic Medicine, Philadelphia;
Neuroscience Administration, Geisinger Health
Systems, Danville, Pennsylvania

SANDEEP S. BHANGOO, MS, MD
Department of Neurosurgery, Hermelin Brain
Tumor Center, Henry Ford Health System,
Detroit, Michigan

NICHOLAS BUTOWSKI, MD
Associate Professor, Director
of Clinical Services, Division of
Neuro-Oncology, Department
of Neurological Surgery,
University of California,
San Francisco, San Francisco,
California

ROUKOZ B. CHAMOUN, MD
Department of Neurosurgery,
Baylor College of Medicine,
Houston, Texas

VINCENT J. CHEUNG, BA
Department of Neurosurgery,
The University of Texas,
MD Anderson Cancer Center,
Houston, Texas

ANTHONY L. D'AMBROSIO, MD
Assistant Professor of Neurological Surgery, Department of Neurological Surgery, Columbia University College of Physicians and Surgeons, New York, New York; Director of Neuro-Oncology, Blumenthal Cancer Center, The Valley Hospital, Ridgewood; Chief, Division of Neurological Surgery, St Joseph's Regional Medical Center, Paterson, New Jersey

FRANCO DEMONTE, MD, FRCSC, FACS
Professor of Neurosurgery and Head and Neck Surgery, Mary Beth Pawelek Chair in Neurosurgery, Department of Neurosurgery, The University of Texas, MD Anderson Cancer Center, Houston, Texas

ROBERT B. DEN, MD
Chief Resident, Department of Radiation Oncology, Thomas Jefferson University, Philadelphia, Pennsylvania

CHAD DEYOUNG, MD
Department of Radiation Oncology, The Valley Hospital, Ridgewood, New Jersey

BENJAMIN D. FOX, MD
Department of Neurosurgery, The University of Texas, MD Anderson Cancer Center, Houston, Texas

MORRIS D. GROVES, MD, JD
Associate Professor, Department of Neuro-Oncology, The University of Texas, MD Anderson Cancer Center, Houston, Texas

STEVEN R. ISAACSON, MD
Department of Radiation Oncology, Columbia University College of Physicians and Surgeons, New York, New York

STEVEN N. KALKANIS, MD
Department of Neurosurgery, Hermelin Brain Tumor Center, Henry Ford Health System, Detroit, Michigan

CHRISTOPHER P. KELLNER, MD
Department of Neurological Surgery, Columbia University College of Physicians and Surgeons, New York, New York

ALEXANDER G. KHANDJI, MD, FACR
Clinical Professor of Radiology, Neuroradiology Division, Radiology Department, Columbia University, New York Presbyterian Medical Center, New York, New York

ANGELA LIGNELLI, MD
Assistant Professor of Radiology, Neuroradiology Division, Radiology Department, Columbia University, New York Presbyterian Medical Center, New York, New York

MARK E. LINSKEY, MD
Departments of Neurosurgery and Neurological Surgery, University of California-Irvine Medical Center, Detroit, Michigan

CHRISTINA A. MEYERS, PhD, ABPP
Professor and Chief, Section of Neuropsychology, Department of Neuro-Oncology, The University of Texas, MD Anderson Cancer Center, Houston, Texas

AKASH J. PATEL, MD
Department of Neurosurgery, The University of Texas, MD Anderson Cancer Center, Houston, Texas

MARYAM RAHMAN, MD, MS
Department of Neurosurgery, University of Florida, Gainesville, Florida

GANESH RAO, MD
Assistant Professor, Department of Neurosurgery, The University of Texas, MD Anderson Cancer Center, Houston, Texas

DIMA SUKI, PhD
Department of Neurosurgery, The University of Texas, MD Anderson Cancer Center, Houston, Texas

STEVEN A. TOMS, MD, MPH
Director, Department of Neurosurgery and Surgical Director, Neuroscience Administration, Geisinger Medical Center, Geisinger Health System, Danville, Philadelphia, Pennsylvania

MARIANA E. WITGERT, PhD
Assistant Professor, Section of Neuropsychology, Department of Neuro-Oncology, The University of Texas, MD Anderson Cancer Center, Houston, Texas

Contents

Epidemiology of Metastatic Brain Tumors   1

Benjamin D. Fox, Vincent J. Cheung, Akash J. Patel, Dima Suki, and Ganesh Rao

> Metastatic tumors are the most common brain tumors in adults, and their incidence is increasing. An accurate understanding of the epidemiology of metastatic brain tumors is useful for health care professionals to allocate appropriate clinical, diagnostic, therapeutic, and research resources. Reported incidences in the literature are derived from epidemiologic population-based studies; clinical studies from surgical, radiological, and autopsy series; and reviews of hospital and clinical medical records. Despite these various sources of information, an accurate incidence of metastatic brain tumors is difficult, and current figures are estimates at best. Here, we review the available data regarding the epidemiology of metastatic brain tumors.

The Molecular Pathobiology of Metastasis to the Brain: A Review   7

Kara D. Beasley and Steven A. Toms

> As the length of survival continues to improve for patients with systemic cancers, the problem of metastases to the chemotherapeutic sanctuary of the central nervous system (CNS) continues to grow. This review focuses on the pathobiology of brain metastasis, attempting to develop a framework for understanding the steps and molecular underpinnings of the metastatic cascade. In this process, cancer cells escape the primary tumor organ, intravasate into blood vessels, survive the hematogenous dissemination to the CNS, arrest in brain capillaries, extravasate, proliferate, and develop angiogenic abilities to succeed as an established metastasis. Each of the steps of the metastatic cascade is dependent on distinct molecular pathways, the identification of which may be exploited in attempting to halt or slow the development of brain metastases.

Review of Imaging Techniques in the Diagnosis and Management of Brain Metastases   15

Angela Lignelli and Alexander G. Khandji

> Brain metastasis is one of the most common diagnoses encountered by neurologists, neurosurgeons, radiologists, and oncologists. The aim of this article is to review imaging modalities used in the diagnosis and follow-up of brain metastases. Through the use of various imaging techniques more accurate preoperative diagnosis and more precise intraoperative planning can be made. Post-treatment evaluation can also be refined through the use of these imaging techniques.

Medical Management of Brain Metastases   27

Nicholas Butowski

> The main objective of treating brain metastases is to improve survival and to reduce symptom burden, preserve function, and enhance quality of life. As such, concurrent local control of existing brain metastases, prevention of future metastasis elsewhere in the brain, and control of the systemic cancer are required. The treatment

modalities used to achieve these aims include surgery, radiation, and medical therapy. This article is devoted to the medical management of brain metastases, namely the role of medical treatments and chemotherapy. Radiation therapy and surgery are discussed in detail elsewhere; however, a brief discussion of all of these modalities is included for the sake of thoroughness.

chemotherapy, and surgery. Surgical resection is reserved for a minority of well-selected patients. The decision to intervene surgically is based on patients' clinical status, the degree of control of systemic disease, the accessibility of the lesion, and the potential morbidity of the procedure. Well-designed trials and evidence-based practice guidelines are not available. The management of these patients largely depends of the experience of the treating medical team.

Leptomeningeal metastasis (LMD) is a lethal complication caused by a variety of cancers, typically developing late in the disease course. It is associated with major neurologic disabilities and short survival. The incidence of LMD may increase because of longer survival of patients who have cancer, and because of the use of newer large-molecule therapies with poor central nervous system penetration. To achieve improved outcomes for patients who have LMD, new treatments need to reach the meninges and cerebrospinal fluid and interact with relevant molecular targets. Some of the agents currently in testing may contribute to this goal. To allow for better outcomes through earlier treatment, advances in diagnosis are needed. By using agents with higher therapeutic indices, in patients with a lower burden of disease (identified earlier with clinical or molecular markers) it should be possible to achieve gradual improvements in outcomes for patients suffering from this devastating disease.

The assessment of neurocognitive function and quality of life (QOL) in patients with brain metastases has become increasingly recognized as an important addition to traditional outcome measures such as length of survival and time to disease progression. Although objective assessment of neurocognitive function using standardized neuropsychological tests is well established, QOL represents a more subjective concept for which no gold standard assessment tool has been identified. Assessment of both neurocognitive function and QOL should involve reliable and valid measures that are sensitive to the cognitive domains and aspects of patient well-being that are most affected by brain metastases and associated treatments. Thorough evaluation of these factors is critical to understanding baseline (ie, pretreatment) cognitive functioning and QOL, monitoring the effects of necessary treatments and allowing comparison of available treatments, informing future treatment decisions, and facilitating the development and implementation of tailored behavioral and pharmacologic interventions that minimize the effect of symptoms on functional well-being.

Contrary to the incidence of primary cancers, the incidence of brain metastasis has been increasing. This increase is likely because of the effects of an aging population, improved neuroimaging surveillance, and better control of systemic cancer, allowing time for brain metastasis to occur. Unlike systemic cancers, for which chemotherapy is the mainstay of treatment, the therapeutic strategies available to treat brain metastasis have traditionally been limited to surgical resection, whole brain radiation therapy, or stereotactic radiosurgery, either individually or in combination. It is important to put the treatment in the context of the prognosis for patients with brain metastases.

The objective of this article is to present a concise summary of the most recent evidence-based guidelines in the management of metastatic brain tumors developed by the American Association of Neurologic Surgeons (AANS), Congress of Neurologic Surgeons (CNS), and the AANS/CNS Joint Section on Tumors in 2010. Target populations include patients with newly diagnosed metastases as well as recurrent or progressive lesions. The roles of radiotherapy, surgical resection, and stereotactic radiosurgery along with combination therapies are reviewed. Other topics include the role of chemotherapy, anticonvulsants, steroids, and investigational therapies.

Neurosurgery Clinics of North America

THE CLINICS ARE NOW AVAILABLE ONLINE!

Access your subscription at:
www.theclinics.com

Neurosurgery Clinics of North America

FORTHCOMING ISSUES

April 2011

Functional Imaging
Peter Black, MD, PhD, and
Alexandra Golby, MD, BWH, Guest Editors

August 2011

Pineal Region Tumors
Jeffrey N. Bruce, MD, and
Andrew Parsa, MD, PhD, Guest Editors

October 2011

Epilepsy
Nicholas Barbaro, MD, and
Edward Chang, MD,
Guest Editors

RECENT ISSUES

October 2010

Minimally Invasive Intracranial Surgery
Michael E. Sughrue, MD, and
Charles Teo, MD, Guest Editors

July 2010

Pediatric Vascular Neurosurgery
Paul Klimo Jr MD, Maj, USAF
Cormac O. Maher, MD, and
Edward R. Smith, MD, Guest Editor

April 2010

Aneurysmal Subarachnoid Hemorrhage
Paul Nyquist, MD, MPH, Rafael Tamargo, MD,
and Rafael J. Tamargo, MD, Guest Editors

RELATED INTEREST

Neuroimaging Clinics August 2010 (Volume 20, Issue 3)
State of the Art Brain Tumor Diagnosis, Imaging, and therapeutics
Meng Law, MD, Guest Editor

THE CLINICS ARE NOW AVAILABLE ONLINE!

Access your subscription at:
www.theclinics.com

Preface

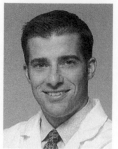
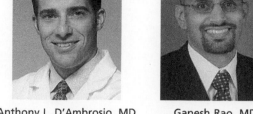

Anthony L. D'Ambrosio, MD   Ganesh Rao, MD

Guest Editors

There is no doubt that the incidence of metastatic cancer to the brain is increasing. As systemic cancer treatments improve, patients are living longer, but they are increasingly prone to develop brain metastases. This is primarily due to the fact that systemic treatments have limited efficacy on metastatic deposits in the brain. In the United States, there are likely to be over 250,000 new cases of brain metastases diagnosed this year. The treatment options available for patients suffering from metastases to the brain are also increasing and are often employed in combination with one another. The evidence supporting the use of these treatments is variable, which can make treatment selection somewhat difficult. This issue of *Neurosurgery Clinics of North America* is intended to cover the pertinent issues regarding metastatic tumors to the brain to assist clinicians from all disciplines in managing these patients. Here, we have assembled a collection of topics we feel will be of value to the neurosurgeon, radiation oncologist, and medical oncologist in selecting treatment for the individual patient.

We are excited to include topics that may not immediately impact the care of patients suffering from a metastatic brain tumor, but will be of interest nonetheless. These include an article on the latest investigational treatments for brain metastases. As medical technology advances at a seemingly exponential rate, many of these new therapeutic strategies will likely find their way into the clinic and/or operating room in short order. Similarly, the understanding of the molecular basis for metastatic disease is also advancing and the article in this issue is intended to introduce these concepts to the reader. Cancer treatments certainly have associated toxicity, and we have devoted an article to help the reader appreciate the quality-of-life issues surrounding the treatments administered to patients. Finally, we are pleased to offer a review of the recently published evidence-based guidelines for the treatment of metastatic brain tumors that were sanctioned by the American Association of Neurological Surgeons and the Congress of Neurological Surgeons. This article provides unique insight into the efficacy of available treatment options in an evidence-based fashion.

We are absolutely indebted to the authors of each article. They are experts in the field and have themselves authored numerous publications regarding the topic of brain metastases. It is our hope that their wisdom imparted on the pages of this issue will provide you with guidance in the management of patients with cancer metastatic to the brain.

Anthony L. D'Ambrosio, MD
Department of Neurological Surgery
Columbia University
College of Physicians and Surgeons
The Neurological Institute
710 West 168th Street, 4th Floor
New York, NY 10032, USA

Ganesh Rao, MD
Department of Neurosurgery
The University of Texas
MD Anderson Cancer Center
1515 Holcombe Boulevard
Houston, TX 77030, USA

E-mail addresses:
ad504@columbia.edu (A.L. D'Ambrosio)
grao@mdanderson.org (G. Rao)

Neurosurg Clin N Am 22 (2011) xi
doi:10.1016/j.nec.2010.09.003
1042-3680/11/$ — see front matter
© 2011 Elsevier Inc. All rights reserved.

Epidemiology of Metastatic Brain Tumors

Benjamin D. Fox, MD, Vincent J. Cheung, BA,
Akash J. Patel, MD, Dima Suki, PhD, Ganesh Rao, MD*

KEYWORDS

- Brain metastasis • Epidemiology • Cancer

Metastatic tumors are the most frequent type of brain tumor in adults. The reported incidence of metastatic brain tumors is increasing but the exact incidence is unknown.[1] This increase in the incidence of metastatic brain tumors is likely because of improved therapeutics resulting in increased survival after initial cancer diagnosis, an aging patient population, and improved diagnostic and screening mechanisms resulting in earlier identification and initiation of treatment in patients with primary cancer.[2,3]

The reported incidence of metastatic brain tumors in the literature is derived from disparate data sources, such as death certificates, cancer registries (from various countries), hospital records, census data, or combinations of these sources. These data are reported in epidemiologic population-based studies or clinical or autopsy series. Each of these studies has its own inherent biases and limitations, and it is difficult to compare these studies because of variations in methodologies used to formulate the epidemiologic characteristics in each study.

As the incidence of metastatic brain tumors increases, so does the need to have a consistent and accurate understanding of the epidemiologic factors associated with these tumors. This information aids health care professionals in planning for the challenges of caring for this population of patients as well as developing preventative measures to decrease the likelihood of metastatic brain disease. The increasing number of patients with metastatic brain tumors places a burden on public health services because these patients strain diagnostic, therapeutic, and research resources.

POPULATION-BASED EPIDEMIOLOGIC STUDIES

Population-based studies are generally considered more accurate and less biased than the more limited clinical or autopsy-based series.[2] Few population-based studies focusing on metastatic tumors of the brain have been reported in the literature, and most of these studies are decades old. Guomundsson[4] published the results of a population-based study performed in Iceland reviewing the incidence of central nervous system (CNS) tumors from 1954 to 1963. The annual incidence of metastatic and primary brain tumors was reported to be 2.8 and 7.8 persons per 100,000 population, respectively. The incidence proportion (defined as the number of patients with metastatic brain tumors by the number of patients with primary brain tumors in that particular population) of metastatic brain tumors in all patients with primary systemic malignancies in that study was less than 20%.[2]

Percy and colleagues[5] reviewed the data from 1935 to 1968 in Rochester, Minnesota, and found a much higher incidence of 11.1 per 100,000 population; however, the study group was mixed, with some patients being diagnosed clinically and others at the time of autopsy (70% of patients) and some with tumors confirmed pathologically

Disclosures: The authors have nothing to disclose.
Department of Neurosurgery, The University of Texas, MD Anderson Cancer Center, 1515 Holcombe Boulevard, Houston, TX 77030, USA
* Corresponding author.
E-mail address: grao@mdanderson.org

Neurosurg Clin N Am 22 (2011) 1–6
doi:10.1016/j.nec.2010.08.007
1042-3680/11/$ — see front matter © 2011 Elsevier Inc. All rights reserved.

and others diagnosed purely based on imaging. A study from Finland evaluating patients with metastatic brain disease from 1975 to 1982 reported the annual incidence of brain metastases and primary brain tumor at 3.4 and 12.3 persons per 100,000 population, respectively; brain metastases comprised 18% of all CNS neoplasms.[6]

In an American survey of intracranial neoplasms, Walker and colleagues[7] used hospital discharge records from 157 hospitals across the United States from 1973 to 1974 and estimated the annual incidence of metastatic and primary brain tumors to be 8.3 and 8.2 persons per 100,000 population, respectively; the incidence proportion of brain metastases was 51%.[2,7] However, only 20% of all the cases reviewed in this study were pathologically verified. Counsell and colleagues[8] identified 122 neuroepithelial primary brain tumors and 214 metastatic brain tumors in their population-based study of the Lothian region of Scotland from 1989 to 1990. They reported a yearly incidence of metastatic brain tumors of 14.3 persons per 100,000 population.

Materljan and colleagues[9] reviewed hospital records in Labin, Croatia, from 1974 to 2001 and found a yearly incidence of metastatic and primary brain tumors to be 9.9 and 11.8 persons per 100,000 population, respectively. Barnholtz-Sloan and colleagues[2] performed a population-based review of the Metropolitan Detroit Cancer Surveillance System from 1973 to 2001 (metro population approximately 4.5 million) and found the incidence proportion of brain metastasis among all patients with systemic malignancies to be 9.6%; however, this study was limited to the major types of cancer (lung, melanoma, breast, renal, colorectal). Smedby and colleagues[10] used the Swedish national population-based health care registers from 1987 to 2006 and found that the annual incidence rate of hospitalization for brain metastases doubled during this period from 7 (in 1987) to 14 (in 2006) persons per 100,000 population. Schouten and colleagues[11] used the Maastricht (Netherlands) Cancer Registry from 1986 to 1995, which covered 95% of the patients in this region, and identified 2724 patients with primary cancer. These patients were followed up until 1998, and 8.5% of them developed subsequent brain metastases, with 72% of the brain metastases occurring within the first year after initial primary cancer diagnosis.

Although population-based epidemiologic studies are considered better than clinical and autopsy-based studies, there are still some notable limitations and biases that are inherent to these types of studies. These defined populations and hospitals being studied are subject to (and limited by) the regional referral patterns, regional access to health care and cancer treatment, and the inherent sampling biases of the pathology of that region. In addition, no 2 population regions have equivalent treatment expertise. Slight variations in clinical aggressiveness in obtaining diagnostic imaging and/or biopsies or even the frequency of autopsies potentially affect the reported incidences of metastatic tumors.

Hospital records, registries, autopsies, and diagnostic imaging studies are subject to the inherent sampling biases, referral patterns, and treatment preferences of that particular region. Studies based on the above-mentioned data sources often underdiagnose the incidence of brain metastases. Many metastatic brain tumors are asymptomatic and are never diagnosed. In addition, patients with end-stage systemic cancer who develop neurologic symptoms near the end of life but are not clinically suitable for treatment given their systemic disease burden are never diagnosed. Up to one-third of all brain metastases are diagnosed at autopsy[12]; however, autopsy rates have significantly declined over the last 3 decades.[13] Furthermore, there is variability in the definition of a metastatic brain tumor in that some studies consider all brain masses in a patient with a history of cancer to be a metastatic brain tumor, whereas other studies include only pathologically verified masses (**Table 1**).

Cancer registries are frequently used in population-based studies to calculate incidence rates. Cancer registries have many advantages over other databases. They are usually confined to a particular state, region, or other defined location; follow all patients with a cancer diagnosis prospectively; record information with regard to status and treatment of cancer and death; and can calculate yearly incidences of cancer diagnoses for the particular population they cover. Smaller population- and hospital-based registries can interact and cooperate with each other and larger registries to cover a larger population size. Cancer registries also have limitations. They do not account for patients living within a defined region who seek medical care outside of the boundaries of the registry. In some American states, the population can be dynamic, which can affect the calculation of an accurate incidence. Further, cancer registries typically focus on and record only the primary cancer histology and primary site of the cancer and frequently do not contain information about metastatic brain tumors. These registries have also been shown to contain the International Classification of Diseases Ninth Revision coding errors and imprecise diagnostic codes.[14] For example, a patient presenting with

Table 1
Population-based epidemiologic studies

Author	Study Year	Location	Brain Metastasis Incidence Rate (Persons per 100,000 Population)
Guomundsson[4]	1954–1963	Iceland	2.8
Percy et al[5]	1935–1968	Rochester, Minnesota	11.1
Fogelholm et al[6]	1975–1982	Finland	3.4
Walker et al[7]	1973–1974	United States	8.3
Counsell et al[8]	1989–1990	Lothian, Scotland	14.3
Materljan et al[9]	1974–2001	Labin, Croatia	9.9
Barnholtz-Sloan et al[2]	1973–2001	Detroit, Michigan	a
Smedby et al[10]	1987–2006	Sweden	7 (1987); 14 (2006)

[a] Study reports incidences as incidence proportions, not incidence rate.

brain metastasis from a primary breast cancer is usually classified as having recurrent breast cancer rather than a separate brain metastasis.[3] For these reasons, population-based and clinical studies can never be exact, and they typically underestimate the true incidence of metastatic brain tumors.

CLINICAL STUDIES

Clinical studies have shown a high degree of variability in their reported incidences of brain metastases and vary significantly in the size and definition of the population being studied. Kawahata and Ohtomo[15] reported on a cohort of elderly patients (median age, 77.5 years; range, 65–88 years) hospitalized with brain tumors in Japan from 1973 to 1987. They identified 322 pathologically confirmed brain tumors with an overall frequency of brain metastases of 5.8%. A study by Grant and colleagues[16] reviewed imaging files, hospital records, and cancer registries in the Lothian region of Scotland from 1989 to 1990, which includes a referral population of 1.2 million patients. They found an annual incidence of intracerebral tumors (both primary and secondary) to be 21.4 per 100,000 population. In their study, 57% and 43% of the patients had metastatic and primary brain tumors, respectively.

Surgical series are an incomplete data source for brain metastasis information because they depend on patients referred for surgery and do not account for the metastases that are not treated surgically. Radiographic series are also incomplete sources to study the epidemiology of brain metastases because routine screening of the brain in patients with asymptomatic cancer is not typically performed except in certain lung cancer types (eg, small cell lung cancer) and they are also subject to the selection bias of referral patterns.[1] Clinical studies based on hospital records are limited by selection bias and often use discharge diagnoses, which can be incorrect or nonspecific. For example, Walker and colleagues[7] found that approximately 10% of these discharge diagnoses lacked specificity using terminology such as probable brain tumor, brain tumor, rule out brain tumor, and suspected brain tumor.

ESTIMATES

Based on earlier and recent population-based studies that typically underestimate the number of metastatic tumors, the incidence of metastatic brain tumors should be between 7 and 14 persons per 100,000 population. The official census data estimates the US population at approximately 310 million,[17] which would correlate with an estimate of 21,651 to 43,301 patients with newly diagnosed brain metastases in the United States in 2010.

Based on autopsy studies, up to one-fourth of patients with a diagnosis of cancer have brain metastases before death.[12,18–20] Based on the annual cancer statistics report, the number of new cases of cancer reported in 2009 was 1,479,350.[21] If one-fourth of those patients develop metastatic brain tumors, 369,837 of these newly diagnosed patients with cancer will develop metastatic brain tumors during their lifetime. Based on the clinical study of Schouten and colleagues[11] (discussed earlier), approximately 70% of these patients develop metastatic brain tumors within the first year after diagnosis, which means at least 258,886 metastatic brain tumors were expected to develop in 2009.

PRIMARY CANCER HISTOLOGY

One of the major factors affecting the incidence of brain metastasis is the histology of the primary cancer.[3] In general, the sources of brain metastases (in descending order) are cancers of the lung, breast, skin, kidney, and gastrointestinal (GI) tract.[22–24] The incidences of brain metastases from other less common primary tumors are reviewed elsewhere.[1,3]

The estimated number of new cases of lung cancer in 2009 was 219,440, with more new cases identified in men than in women; however, the incidence has been increasing in women in recent years.[21] Lung cancer is generally accepted as the most frequent source of metastatic brain tumors. It accounts for 30% to 60% of all brain metastases and occurs in 17% to 65% of patients with primary lung cancer.[1,3] Of the various types of lung cancer, small cell lung cancer and adenocarcinoma are the most commonly identified sources of brain metastases. Lung cancer frequently presents with brain metastases causing the first symptoms prompting further workup, ultimately resulting in the diagnosis of lung cancer. The median interval between initial cancer diagnosis and identification of a metastatic brain tumor is shortest for lung cancer and ranges from 2 to 9 months,[3] with 91% of patients with lung cancer being diagnosed with brain metastases within 1 year of initial diagnosis.[11]

The estimated number of new cases of breast cancer in 2009 was 192,370.[21] Breast cancer is typically the most common cause of brain metastasis in women. It accounts for 5% to 30% of all metastatic brain tumors in women and occurs in up to 30% of women with primary breast cancer.[3,25,26] In contrast to lung cancer, breast cancer brain metastases are commonly a late occurrence, with a median interval of 2 to 3 years between initial cancer diagnosis and identification of a metastatic brain tumor.[3,25]

The incidence of primary malignant melanoma has been increasing over the last decade. The estimated number of new cases of primary malignant melanoma in 2009 was 68,720, with more new cases identified in men than in women.[21] Of all metastatic brain tumors, melanoma accounts for 5% to 21% and has been reported as having the highest propensity to metastasize to the brain.[3,19,27–29] Approximately 37% of patients with stage IV melanoma develop brain metastases, and autopsy series report an incidence as high as 90% (range, 12%–90%).[3,29] Metastases typically occur late, with the median interval of 1 to 3 years between initial cancer diagnosis and identification of a metastatic brain tumor and

multiple brain metastases being typical of this histology.[3,29] Metastatic melanoma to the brain is typically associated with a poorer prognosis than other brain metastases.[30]

The estimated number of new cases of kidney cancer (renal cell carcinoma) in 2009 was 57,760, with more new cases identified in men than in women.[21] The incidence proportion of metastatic brain tumors from renal cancer in patients with primary renal tumors ranges from 5.5% to 11%.[2,11,31,32] The median interval between initial cancer diagnosis and identification of a metastatic renal brain tumor is approximately 1 to 2 years.[3]

The estimated number of new cases of GI cancer in 2009 was 146,970, with a few more new cases identified in men than in women.[21] Colorectal cancers account for 1.4% to 4.8% of all metastatic brain tumors, and approximately 10% of patients with stage IV colorectal cancer have brain metastases.[3,11,33–36] The median interval between initial GI cancer diagnosis and identification of a metastatic brain tumor is approximately 2 to 3 years.[3]

OTHER FACTORS

Other factors that have been reported to affect the incidence of brain metastases are the stage of the primary cancer, age, sex, and race.[2,3] Barnholtz-Sloan and colleagues[2] reported that there was a statistically significant trend of increased incidence proportion of metastatic brain tumors with increasing SEER (Surveillance, Epidemiology, and End Results) stage of all primary cancers (lung, breast, melanoma, renal, GI) included in their study. The primary cancer with the highest incidence proportion of brain metastasis was distant-stage melanoma, which correlates with previous studies reporting a high propensity for melanoma to metastasize to the brain. In patients with breast cancer, stage-related factors that have been shown to be associated with an increased risk of brain metastases are lymph node status, tumor grade, and primary tumor size.[37–40]

Age at diagnosis of primary cancer has a significant effect on the incidence of brain metastases. Metastatic brain tumors are more common in adults than in children, with the highest incidence in general occurring in patients aged 50 to 80 years.[20,33,41] However, the peak ages for brain metastases from breast cancer seem to be lower than the peak ages for other primary pathologies. In a population-based assessment of brain metastases in the Metropolitan Detroit Cancer Surveillance System, the peak incidence proportion for breast cancer brain metastases was during the third decade (for lung cancer, it was during the fourth decade). The median age of patients with breast cancer brain metastases is 5 years less than that of patients without brain metastases.[25]

Although the absolute number of patients with brain metastases is higher in the older population with cancer, younger adult patients with cancer may have a higher proportion of brain metastasis, which may be because of biologic differences and a more aggressive cancer phenotype in these younger adult patients.[3,18,20,42,43] The most common brain metastases in children are leukemia and lymphoma.[20] When considering only solid tumor primary cancers, osteogenic sarcoma, rhabdomyosarcoma, and Ewing sarcoma are the most common primary cancers causing brain metastases.[41] In children with solid primary tumors, brain metastases occur in 4% to 13% of the patients.[22,41,44,45]

A few studies have reported differences in incidences of brain metastases based on gender[2,7]; however, most have not.[3] Lung cancer and breast cancer are the most common sources of brain metastases in men and women, respectively. However, the incidence of primary lung cancer as well as metastases is increasing in women.[2] The incidence of primary malignant melanoma and, subsequently, melanoma brain metastases is increasing in men.[2]

Barnholtz-Sloan and colleagues[2] found an increased incidence proportion of breast cancer and melanoma metastases in African American patients compared with all other patients. The finding that race affects the incidence of brain metastases may be related to the specific population that was studied in the metropolitan Detroit area. Most studies have not reported race as a factor affecting the incidence of brain metastases.

SUMMARY

The exact incidence of metastatic brain tumors is unknown, and the reported incidences in the literature are estimates at best. Epidemiologic population-based studies, clinical studies, and autopsy series have limitations; however, it is clear that metastatic brain tumors are the most frequent type of brain tumor in adults and their incidence is significantly higher than that of primary brain tumors. Primary cancer histology, age at diagnosis, and primary tumor stage are significant factors that affect the epidemiology of metastatic brain disease.

REFERENCES

1. Gavrilovic IT, Posner JB. Brain metastases: epidemiology and pathophysiology. J Neurooncol 2005; 75:5.

2. Barnholtz-Sloan JS, Sloan AE, Davis FG, et al. Incidence proportions of brain metastases in patients diagnosed (1973 to 2001) in the Metropolitan Detroit Cancer Surveillance System. J Clin Oncol 2004;22:2865.

3. Suki D. The epidemiology of brain metastasis. In: Sawaya R, editor. Intracranial metastases: current management strategies. Malden (MA): Blackwell; 2004. p. 20.

4. Guomundsson KR. A survey of tumors of the central nervous system in Iceland during the 10-year period 1954–1963. Acta Neurol Scand 1970;46:538.

5. Percy AK, Elveback LR, Okazaki H, et al. Neoplasms of the central nervous system. Epidemiologic considerations. Neurology 1972;22(1):40–8.

6. Fogelholm R, Uutela T, Murros K. Epidemiology of central nervous system neoplasms. A regional survey in Central Finland. Acta Neurol Scand 1984; 69:129.

7. Walker AE, Robins M, Weinfeld FD. Epidemiology of brain tumors: the national survey of intracranial neoplasms. Neurology 1985;35:219.

8. Counsell CE, Collie DA, Grant R. Incidence of intracranial tumours in the Lothian region of Scotland, 1989–1990. J Neurol Neurosurg Psychiatr 1996; 61:143.

9. Materljan E, Materljan B, Sepcic J, et al. Epidemiology of central nervous system tumors in Labin area, Croatia, 1974–2001. Croat Med J 2004;45: 206.

10. Smedby KE, Brandt L, Backlund ML, et al. Brain metastases admissions in Sweden between 1987 and 2006. Br J Cancer 2009;101:1919.

11. Schouten LJ, Rutten J, Huveneers HA, et al. Incidence of brain metastases in a cohort of patients with carcinoma of the breast, colon, kidney, and lung and melanoma. Cancer 2002;94:2698.

12. Posner JB, Chernik NL. Intracranial metastases from systemic cancer. Adv Neurol 1978;19:579.

13. Shojania KG, Burton EC, McDonald KM, et al. Changes in rates of autopsy-detected diagnostic errors over time: a systematic review. JAMA 2003; 289:2849.

14. Counsell CE, Collie DA, Grant R. Limitations of using a cancer registry to identify incident primary intracranial tumours. J Neurol Neurosurg Psychiatr 1997;63:94.

15. Kawahata N, Ohtomo E. [Metastatic brain tumor in the elderly]. Rinsho Shinkeigaku 1989;29:1106 [in Japanese].

16. Grant R, Whittle IR, Collie DA, et al. Referral pattern and management of patients with malignant brain tumours in South East Scotland. Health Bull (Edinb) 1996;54:212.

17. Availabe at: www.census.gov. Accessed May 13, 2010.

18. Aronson SM, Garcia JH, Aronson BE. Metastatic neoplasms of the brain: their frequency in relation to age. Cancer 1964;17:558.

19. Chason JL, Walker FB, Landers JW. Metastatic carcinoma in the central nervous system and dorsal root ganglia. A prospective autopsy study. Cancer 1963;16:781.

20. Takakura K, Sano K, Hojo S, et al. Metastatic tumors of the central nervous system. Tokyo: Igaku-Shoin; 1983.

21. Jemal A, Siegel R, Ward E, et al. Cancer statistics, 2009. CA Cancer J Clin 2009;59:225.

22. Posner JB. Brain metastases: 1995. A brief review. J Neurooncol 1996;27:287.

23. Sawaya R, Bindal R, Lang F, et al. Metastatic brain tumors. In: Kaye E, editor. Brain tumors: an encyclopedic approach. 2nd edition. London: Churchill Livingstone; 2001. p. 999.

24. Weinberg JS, Lang FF, Sawaya R. Surgical management of brain metastases. Curr Oncol Rep 2001;3:476.

25. Cheng X, Hung MC. Breast cancer brain metastases. Cancer Metastasis Rev 2007;26:635.

26. Graesslin O, Abdulkarim BS, Coutant C, et al. Nomogram to predict subsequent brain metastasis in patients with metastatic breast cancer. J Clin Oncol 2010;28:2032.

27. Amer MH, Al-Sarraf M, Baker LH, et al. Malignant melanoma and central nervous system metastases: incidence, diagnosis, treatment and survival. Cancer 1978;42:660.

28. Pickren JW, Lopez G, Tsukada Y, et al. Brain metastases: an autopsy study. Cancer Treat Symposia 1983;2:295.

29. Sloan AE, Nock CJ, Einstein DB. Diagnosis and treatment of melanoma brain metastasis: a literature review. Cancer Control 2009;16:248.

30. Douglas JG, Margolin K. The treatment of brain metastases from malignant melanoma. Semin Oncol 2002;29:518.

31. Harada Y, Nonomura N, Kondo M, et al. Clinical study of brain metastasis of renal cell carcinoma. Eur Urol 1999;36:230.

32. Saitoh H. Distant metastasis of renal adenocarcinoma. Cancer 1981;48:1487.

33. Graf AH, Buchberger W, Langmayr H, et al. Site preference of metastatic tumours of the brain. Virchows Arch A Pathol Anat Histopathol 1988;412:493.

34. Ishikura A, Hunaki N, Watanabe K. [Brain metastases of colorectal cancer—a case report]. Gan No Rinsho 1987;33:188 [in Japanese].

35. Patanaphan V, Salazar OM. Colorectal cancer: metastatic patterns and prognosis. South Med J 1993;86:38.

36. Welch JP, Donaldson GA. The clinical correlation of an autopsy study of recurrent colorectal cancer. Ann Surg 1979;189:496.

37. Gabos Z, Sinha R, Hanson J, et al. Prognostic significance of human epidermal growth factor receptor positivity for the development of brain metastasis after newly diagnosed breast cancer. J Clin Oncol 2006;24:5658.

38. Hicks DG, Short SM, Prescott NL, et al. Breast cancers with brain metastases are more likely to be estrogen receptor negative, express the basal cytokeratin CK5/6, and overexpress HER2 or EGFR. Am J Surg Pathol 2006;30:1097.

39. Pestalozzi BC, Zahrieh D, Price KN, et al. Identifying breast cancer patients at risk for central nervous system (CNS) metastases in trials of the International Breast Cancer Study Group (IBCSG). Ann Oncol 2006;17:935.

40. Tham YL, Sexton K, Kramer R, et al. Primary breast cancer phenotypes associated with propensity for central nervous system metastases. Cancer 2006; 107:696.

41. Graus F, Walker RW, Allen JC. Brain metastases in children. J Pediatr 1983;103:558.

42. de la Monte SM, Hutchins GM, Moore GW. Influence of age on the metastatic behavior of breast carcinoma. Hum Pathol 1988;19:529.

43. Sorensen JB, Hansen HH, Hansen M, et al. Brain metastases in adenocarcinoma of the lung: frequency, risk groups, and prognosis. J Clin Oncol 1988;6:1474.

44. Tasdemiroglu E, Patchell RA. Cerebral metastases in childhood malignancies. Acta Neurochir (Wien) 1997;139:182.

45. Vannucci RC, Baten M. Cerebral metastatic disease in childhood. Neurology 1974;24:981.

The Molecular Pathobiology of Metastasis to the Brain: A Review

Kara D. Beasley, DO, MBe[a,b,c], Steven A. Toms, MD, MPH[c,d],*

KEYWORDS

- Brain metastasis • Molecular biology • Genetics
- Pathobiology

The issue of brain metastasis is an increasing problem for oncologists and neurosurgeons. Although improved cancer therapies have increased the survival rates of many cancers, brain metastases continue to have poor overall survival rates. Thus, there continues to be a need for the discovery of new and different targets to prevent a tumor from escaping from its site of origin, migrating to the brain, and continuing to proliferate at distant sites. This process is commonly referred to as the metastatic cascade and is highly dependent on a multitude of cellular processes, each of which must be present and functioning in order for successful metastasis (Appendix 1).

The incidence of brain metastasis is unknown, but estimates range from 140,000 to 170,000 new cases per year.[1] It is well known that certain cancers preferentially metastasize to the brain, specifically lung (50%–60%), breast (15%–20%), melanoma (5%–10%), and renal and colon cancers (4%–6%).[2,3] Twenty to 30% of all patients who have breast cancer eventually develop central nervous system (CNS) metastasis.[1] The treatment of metastasis to the brain is further complicated by the unique characteristics of the brain. The blood-brain barrier (BBB), with its tight junctions and lack of lymphatic drainage, makes the delivery of chemotherapeutic agents difficult and represents a therapeutic haven from chemotherapy. In addition, the microenvironment of the brain parenchyma is unique. The interstitial fluid of the brain is high in chloride, which may make the parenchyma a hostile environment to many metastatic clones and favor clones of neuroepithelial origin, such as small-cell carcinoma of the lung or melanoma.

This article reviews the known pathobiologic components of the ability of primary tumors to metastasize at each stage of the metastatic cascade. The promoters, contributors, and inhibitors of the cascade are numerous and may become overwhelming without an organizational structure within which to arrange the alphabet soup of chemicals and genes that are involved in this process. By examining the genetic and pathobiologic characteristics of the process in this matter, we hope to create a more structured platform for understanding this complex process that allows the clinician to create a framework of current therapeutics and possible future research.

ESCAPE/INTRAVASATION

For a primary tumor to metastasize to a secondary site, it must break free from the primary tumor and enter the vasculature. Although many of the

The authors have nothing to disclose.
[a] Geisinger Medical Center, 100 North Academy Avenue, MC 14-5, Danville, PA 17821, USA
[b] Philadelphia College of Osteopathic Medicine, Philadelphia, PA, USA
[c] Neuroscience Administration, MC 14-5, Geisinger Health Systems, 100 North Academy Avenue, Danville, PA 17822, USA
[d] Neuroscience Administration, Geisinger Medical Center, Danville, PA, USA
* Corresponding author. Neuroscience Administration, MC 14-5, Geisinger Health Systems, 100 North Academy Avenue, Danville, PA 17822.
E-mail address: satoms@geisinger.edu

Neurosurg Clin N Am 22 (2011) 7–14
doi:10.1016/j.nec.2010.08.009
1042-3680/11/$ – see front matter © 2011 Elsevier Inc. All rights reserved.

molecular processes discussed later are active at both the escape and extravasation/proliferation stages, they are first encountered within the cascade early on and so are addressed in this section.

The E-cadherin-catenin complex is vital for the maintenance of both normal and tumoral cytoarchitecture as well as a necessary mediator of cell-cell adhesion. In the metastatic escape of a tumor, clone cells have reduced intercellular adhesion and disordered cytoarchitecture, and are thus prone to separation from the primary tumor mass. These clones are then free to invade both locally as well as to continue on to intravasation and further progress in the cascade.[4] Decreased expression of the E-cadherin-catenin complex has been correlated with invasion, metastasis, and unfavorable prognosis.[5] In addition, Shabani and colleagues[6] established a correlation between E-cadherin-catenin complex expression and an increased mindbomb homolog 1 (MIB1) index in metastatic adenocarcinoma.

Another family of adhesion and signaling receptor proteins are the integrins. They mediate both cell migration and tumor invasion via the triggering of multiple signal transduction pathways. They are therefore vital in the complex cascade of regulation of such processes as gene expression, growth control, cytoskeletal architecture, and apoptosis. In an animal model of human nonsmall-cell lung cancer (NSCLC), blocking of the $\alpha_3\beta_1$-integrin significantly decreased brain metastasis.[7] Researchers at Oxford showed that the blockage of the β_1-integrin subunit prevented tumor cell adhesion to the vascular basement membrane (VBM) and attenuated metastasis establishment and growth in vivo.[8] Furthermore, focal adhesion kinase (FAK) is known to be a key mediator in integrin signaling and therefore is believed to play a role in metastatic migration and proliferation. Dephosphorylation and therefore the inhibition of FAK at the Y397 locus via activated oncogene (rat sarcoma) has been shown to promote tumor migration via the facilitation of focal adhesion turnover at the leading edge of tumor cells.[9,10]

Another aspect of the ability of a tumor cell to escape the local site is its ability to break down or functionally remodel the extracellular matrix (ECM). Degradation of the ECM via proteolytic enzymes is believed to clear a pathway for invasion. This proteolytic activity has been located on the cell membrane at the advancing edge of invading tumor cells.[11,12] The ECM proteolysis may also release factors that promote cell proliferation and angiogenesis for contribution to later steps in the cascade. Neurotrophins (NTs) are known to promote brain invasion via enhancing the production of the ECM proteolytic enzyme heparinase. Heparinase is an endo-β-D-glucuronidase that cleaves the heparin sulfate chains of the ECM. It is the dominant mammalian heparin sulfate degradative enzyme[13] and is known to destroy both the ECM and the BBB.[4] NTs have been found at the tumor-brain interface of melanoma,[14] and there are reports of the p75 NT receptor functioning as a molecular determinant for brain metastasis.[15]

Next on the list of molecular degraders of the ECM are the plasminogen activators and their inhibitors. Plasmin is a tumor-associated serine protease activated by urokinase-type plasminogen activator (uPA). The production and release of uPA has been well documented in human cancers.[15] The uPA binds to the receptor uPA-R (CD87), the activity of which is regulated by the action of plasminogen activator inhibitor type 1 and 2 (PAI-1/2) on the cell membrane and causes urokinase to convert plasminogen to plasmin. The proteolytic activity of plasmin then degrades components of the ECM including fibrin, fibronectin, proteoglycans, and laminin. Further, plasmin activates other proteolytic enzymes, with resultant local invasion and migration.[4] As far back as 1994, researchers have found that there are high levels of uPA in metastatic tumors, that uPA correlates with necrosis and edema, and that there is an inverse correlation with levels of uPA of a tumor and survival. In addition, high levels of uPA and absent tissue plasminogen activator correlate with aggressiveness and decreased survival.[16]

The matrix metalloproteases (MMPs) are a family of 20 proteolytic enzymes that have also been well established as functioning to degrade the ECM in metastasis. Their expression is regulated via cytokines, and the ECM metalloprotease inducer is found on the surface of tumor cells. With induction and stimulation, there is an ECM breakdown and a tumor cell migration. MMP activity is known to correlate with invasiveness, metastasis, and poor prognosis.[17] One study found that MMP-2 is present in all metastatic brain tumors tested regardless of the site of origin and that the level of activity inversely correlated with survival.[18] However, although MMP-9 was found by Arnold and colleagues[19] to be upregulated in all brain metastases and primary brain tumors, there was an inability to correlate upregulation with survival. The tissue inhibitor of metalloprotease 1 (TIMP-1) overexpression in a murine model was shown to reduce the incidence of brain metastasis by 75% compared with wild type, showing that inhibitors of MMPs suppress brain metastasis.[20]

The properties of the tumor cell membranes may contribute to the local invasiveness and migratory capability of tumor clones. In a study on brain-specific breast cancer metastasis, Khaitan and colleagues[21] showed that the increased expression of KCNMA1, the gene that encodes for the pore-forming α-subunit of the large-conductance calcium and voltage-activated potassium channel big-conductance type potassium channel that is known to be upregulated in breast cancer, has led to greater invasiveness and transendothelial migration.[21] Furthermore, there has been increased interest in the scientific role of the family of membrane proteins known as aquaporins. Among their many functional roles, aquaporins are known to facilitate tumor migration, as seen in aquaporin-dependent tumor angiogenesis and metastasis via a mechanism of facilitated water transport in the lamellipodia of migrating cells.[22]

Several known tumor-suppressor genes that function at the level of escape and migration/intravasation are worth exploring. The best known of these is the KISS-1 gene on chromosome 1. KISS-1 encodes metastin, which is a ligand of the orphan G protein couples receptor hOT7T175. Lee and colleagues[23] found that the forced expression of KISS-1 suppressed both melanoma and breast metastasis. Other investigators have found an inverse correlation between KISS-1 expression and melanoma progression.[24]

KAI1 (CD82) is another tumor-suppressor gene on chromosome 11p11.2. KAI1 functions to regulate adhesion, migration, growth, and differentiation of tumor cell lines. It has been found to have an inverse correlation with prostate progression[25] as well as breast[26,27] and melanoma metastasis.[28] In addition, KAI1 is known to be associated with the epidermal growth factor receptor (EGFR), discussed later in this article, and is believed to affect the Rho GTPase pathway,[29] resulting in suppression of lamellipodia formation and migration.[30]

The tumor suppressor, Drg-1 methylated inhibition, has been found to inhibit both liver metastasis and colorectal carcinoma invasion.[31] Overexpression of this gene has been linked to resistance to ironectan chemotherapy.[32] In a murine model of breast cancer metastasis, the Notch signaling pathway was found to be activated via increased Jag2 mRNA, creating a cell line that was both more migratory and more invasive in collagen assays. In addition, inactivation of the Notch pathway significantly decreased the migratory and invasive activity of the studied cell lines.[33]

ARREST/EXTRAVASATION

The next series of steps in the metastatic cascade involve a complex set of interactions that allow the tumor clones that have invaded the blood stream to arrest at a secondary site and extravasate from the vasculature to establish a metastasis in a new organ. The clones must then survive and proliferate at the secondary site. Although the exact causes of arrest and proliferation at specific sites have not been completely elucidated, one theory is that there are direct neurotropic interactions between tumor clones and the brain along with yet undiscovered brain-specific homing capacity within the tumor cells that result in brain metastasis. Carbonell and colleagues[8] described a process termed vascular cooption, whereby 95% of micrometastasis are observed to grow along the exterior of preexisting vessels before any overt metastatic tumor is detected. The VBM tumor cell interaction is adhesive in nature. This interaction implied that the VBM is the soil for brain metastasis rather than a previously theorized neurotropism.[8] With the VBM as a substrate, tumor cells are able to infiltrate the brain parenchyma. Saito and colleagues[34] showed that the pia-glial membrane, present along the external surface of blood vessels, serves as a scaffold for metastatic tumor cells spreading in an angiocentric pattern, which furthers the hypothesis of a perivascular soil.

A biologic model for metastatic tumor cells describes how they function like macrophages both within the vasculature and during extravasation in a mouse model of CNS metastasis. In this model, the tumor cells expressed multiple properties of macrophages that included morphologic appearance, surface adhesion, phagocytosis, total lipid composition, and expression of CD11b, Iba1, F4/80, CD68, CD45, and CXCR (all genes specifically expressed by macrophages).[35] It is possible that by expressing these molecules, the metastases can mimic macrophages and escape the immune system while traveling through the vascular system.

The exact mechanisms by which cancer cells pass through the BBB is unknown. However, recently, 3 genes that mediate brain-specific breast metastasis have been described. Cyclooxygenase 2 (COX-2, also known as PTGS-2) as well as the EGFR ligand, heparin-binding epidermal growth factor have been linked to metastasis to the lung as well as to the brain. In addition, these genes function to assist extravasation through nonfenestrated capillaries and enhance colonization.[36] The $\alpha_{2,6}$-sialyltransferase ST6GALNAC5 is normally restricted to the brain and when expressed by breast cancer cells, enhances their adhesion to brain endothelium and their passage through the BBB via cell surface glycosylation.[36]

The chemokine/receptor system, CXCL12/CXCR4, and the recently discovered alternate receptor, CXCR7, function in the homing of neoplastic cells from the primary site to the target site in metastatic disease. In a study of 56 patients with metastatic lesions to the brain from differing primary sites, Salmaggi and colleagues[37] found that CXCL12 was expressed in tumor cells and tumor vessels, and this expression correlated with shorter survival. In addition, the CXCR7 was expressed by tumor cells as well as by the adjacent brain, and the CXCR4 was present in all samples with a nuclear pattern. However, the expression of these receptors did not correlate with survival. Thus, the expression of CXCL12 may indicate aggressiveness of brain-specific metastasis.[37] Another recently described mediator of organ-specific breast cancer metastasis is the expression of heat-shock protein (HSP27). HSP27 is a chaperone of the small heat-shock protein (sHSP) family. Researchers have been able to associate the expression of HSP27 in brain-specific breast cancer metastatic cell lines with the 36/67-laminin receptor. HSP27 created clusters of chaperone and cochaperone proteins that facilitate brain-specific metastasis. In addition, HSP27 associated these chaperone clusters through kinases to a group of filament proteins that may assist in organ-specific homing.[38]

The wingless integration gene (WNT) and T-cell factor (TCF) pathway, WNT/TCF pathway, and its target genes, homeobox B9 and lymphoid-enhancing factor 1, are mediators of brain-specific chemotactic invasion and colony outgrowth in lung adenocarcinoma. Hyperactivity of this pathway is present in metastatic subpopulations of adenocarcinoma cells. Decreases in the activity of TCF attenuates the ability of the cells to form brain and bone metastasis, which indicates their contribution to brain-specific metastatic of lung adenocarcinoma lesions.[39]

Adding to the list of brain-specific contributors to metastasis, Zhang and colleagues[40] described another brain-specific molecular determinant for metastasis of melanoma in a murine model. The investigators found that the transforming growth factor β2 (TGFβ2) was highly expressed in brain-specific murine melanoma cell lines. After transfection of the TGFβ2 gene into another cell line, an increase was noted in the production of microscopic metastatic lesions to brain parenchyma.[40]

Adhesion of neoplastic cells to the endothelium of metastatic sites via a hyaluronate matrix ligand is mediated by CD44 on chromosome 11p11.2.

CD44 encodes a membrane glycoprotein that acts as a receptor for hyaluronic acid and osteopontin.[41–43] CD44 can be downregulated via DNA methylation,[44] and such downregulation has been correlated with increased tumor grade. In addition, upregulation occurs in 48% of brain metastases studied, especially thyroid, melanoma, and breast.[45] Primary brain tumors express the standard form of CD44, whereas metastatic lesions almost exclusively express the only splicing variant of the gene product, providing clinicians with a possible tumor marker for metastatic potential.[46]

Invasion of brain parenchyma is mediated by the tumor-suppressor gene phosphate and tensin homolog deleted on chromosome 10 (PTEN) or mutated in multiple advance cancers (MMAC1). The PTEN/MMAC gene product and the cytoskeletal protein tensin are similar and interact with actin filaments at focal cell adhesions that inhibit cell migration in the functioning gene, whereas, in an antisense mutation, migration was enhanced.[47–49] In lung cancer metastasis, 25% of the genes had an inactivating mutation, suggesting that migration and metastatic progression are inhibited by the normally functioning gene.[50]

Angiogenesis and Metastatic Clone Proliferation

Tumor angiogenesis is an important aspect of the ability of a neoplastic population to survive and grow at a secondary site. Failure of vascular growth ultimately restricts the tumor mass to 0.2 mm or to the limits of tissue diffusion distance.[51] There seems to be a balanced interplay of proangiogenic and antiangiogenic factors.[4] Much research has been devoted in recent years to the elucidation of these angiogenic factors as a target for tumor treatment.

The most commonly recognized of these neoplastic angiogenic factors is vascular endothelial growth factor (VEGF). Kim and colleagues[52] found that VEGF expression plays a role in the ability of breast cancer cells to metastasize, and that the inhibition of VEGF, via a receptor tyrosine kinase inhibitor, reduces tumor-induced angiogenesis and restricted tumor growth. SSecks (Src-suppressed C kinase substrate) is known to decrease the expression of VEGF via reduction of angiogenesis. It also stimulates the expression of the proangiogenic molecule angiopoietin 1 and may regulate the brain angiogenesis and tight junction formation, therefore regulating BBB differentiation and contributing to angiogenesis.[53]

Yet another angiogenic regulator is a member of the previously mentioned MMP family, the

MMP-9/gelatinaseB complex, that may contribute to the switch from vascular quiescence to angiogenesis.[4,54] PAI-1, the uPA cell-surface receptor mentioned earlier, is often localized to the proliferating vessels in brain metastasis and therefore may also play a role in angiogenesis.[55] Plexin D1 expression in tumor versus nonneoplastic vasculature was explored to determine if plexin D1 is unique to tumor cells and vasculature, thus participating in tumor angiogenesis. Plexin D1 was found to be expressed in neoplastic cells as well as tumor vasculature, whereas its expression in nonneoplastic tissue was restricted to a small subset of activated macrophages, suggesting that plexin D1 may play a significant role in tumor angiogenesis.[56]

A significant contributor to the secondary-site tumor for growth potential in breast cancer is overexpression of hexokinase 2 (HK2), which plays a key role in glucose metabolism and apoptosis. Researchers at the National Cancer Institute found that both mRNA and protein levels of HK2 were increased in brain metastatic derivative cell lines compared with the parental cell line in vitro. In addition, these investigators found that the knockdown of expression reduced cell proliferation, implying that the gene contributes to the proliferation and growth of breast cancer metastasis. They showed that increased expression was associated with poor survival after craniotomy.[57]

At least 2 tumor-suppressor genes that function at the proliferation level of the metastatic cascade have been described. The first gene, NM23, regulates cell growth by encoding for a nucleotide diphosphate protein kinase that interacts with menin, which is a putative tumor suppressor encoded by the gene MEN1.[58] NM23 is believed to reduce signal transduction and thereby decrease anchorage-independent colonization, invasion, and motility.[59] In melanoma, decreased expression is correlated with increased brain metastasis.[60] The second described tumor-suppressor gene, BrMS1, localizes to chromosome 11 in melanoma and breast cancers. BrMS1 prevents disseminated tumor cell growth by restoring the normal gap junction phenotype and maintaining cell-to-cell communication in the primary tumor.[61] Seraj and colleagues[62] found an inverse correlation between the expression of BrMS1 and the metastatic potential in melanoma.

Cascade Nonspecific Metastatic Contributors

Certain molecular contributions cannot be attributed to a specific step in the cascade either because they are active at every level, or, as in most cases, their true function is yet to be discovered. These molecular entities are on the forefront of cancer science and are worth addressing. Zeb-1, the zinc finger E-box homeobox transcription factor, is overexpressed in metastatic cancers. This overexpression leads to epithelial-mesenchymal transition and increased metastasis. The mutation of this gene has been shown to decrease proliferation of progenitor cells in mutant mice. This mutation may be a target for metastatic prevention at the progenitor level.[63]

Several other genetic markers have been located that pertain to metastasis in particular. A deletion of the 4q arm in lung (both small- and nonsmall-cell) metastasis to the brain and bone has been documented.[64] In addition, in NSCLC, the overexpression of 3 genes, CDH2 (N-cadherin), KIFC1, and FALZ, was highly predictive of metastasis to the brain in early and advanced lung cancer. Therefore, these genes may be used to predict a high risk of metastasis early in the diagnosis.[65] In prostate cancer, increased expression of KLF6-SV1, the Kruppel-like factor tumor-suppressor gene, predicted poorer survival and correlated with increased metastasis to lymph, brain, and bone.[66] Overexpression of homeoprotein Six-1, a transcriptional regulator, increased TGFβ signaling, and metastasis in breast cancer, with significantly shortened relapse times.[67] These genes are important in the understanding of the metastatic cascade as well as for further research.

SUMMARY

The process by which a tumor cell leaves its primary tumor, travels through the vasculature, and ends up in the brain to proliferate and cause neurologic injury and even death is complex. By understanding as many of the molecular and genetic factors that contribute to the cascade, we are better equipped to target brain metastases using a multitude of strategies. Knowledge of the metastatic process may lead to better detection and treatment of brain metastases. However, our goal is to use this knowledge to prevent the formation of brain metastases in patients with cancer.

APPENDIX 1: GENE SUMMARY

BrMS1: breast cancer metastasis suppressor 1
CXCL12/CXCR4: chemokine/receptor system involved in stem-cell differentiation
CXCR7: alternate receptor to CXCL12
CD11b: cluster of differentiation molecule 11b
CD45: cluster of differentiation 45
CD44: cluster of differentiation 44
CD68: cluster of differentiation 68
CD87: uPA binds to the receptor uPA-R

CDH2: (neutral cadherin [N-cadherin], when overexpressed with FALZ and KIFC1 genes, predicts metastasis to brain

COX-2: cyclooxygenase 2 (also known as PTGS-2)

CXCR: chemokine receptor

Drg-1: differentiation-related, putative metastatic suppressor gene

F4/80: transmembrane protein present on cell surface of mouse

FALZ: overexpressed with CDH2 and KIFC1 genes, predicts metastasis to the brain

HK2: hexokinase 2

HOXB9: homeobox B9

HSP27: heat-shock protein

Iba1: ionized calcium-binding adaptor molecule 1

KAI1 (CD82) gene: tumor-suppressor gene

KCNMA1: tumor-suppressor gene

KIFC1: overexpressed with CDH2 and FALZ genes predicts metastasis to brain

KISS-1: gene that encodes metastin

KLF6-SV1: Kruppel-like factor tumor-suppressor gene

LEF1: lymphoid-enhancing factor 1

MEN1: multiple endocrine neoplasia type 1

MMAC1: mutated in multiple advanced cancers

NM23: metastasis-suppressor gene also known as NDP kinase

Plexin D1: protein that in humans is encoded by the PLXND1 gene

PTEN: phosphatase and tensin homolog located on chromosome 10 (alternatively called MMAC1: mutated in multiple advanced cancers)

Ras: oncogene (rat sarcoma) gene

SSecks-Src: suppressed C kinase substrate

Six-1: homeoprotein transcriptional regulator

ST6GALNAC5: $\alpha_{2,6}$-sialyltransferase that modifies proteins involved in cell-cell interactions

WNT: wingless integration gene

Zeb-1: zinc finger E-box-binding homeobox 1

REFERENCES

1. Horner MJ, Ries LAG, Krapcho M, et al, editors. SEER cancer statistics review, 1975-2006. Available at: http://seer.cancer.gov/csr/1975_2006/index.html. Accessed March 25, 2010.
2. Landis SH, Murray T, Bolden S, et al. Cancer statistics, 1999. CA Cancer J Clin 1999;49(1):8–31.
3. Patchell RA. The management of brain metastases. Cancer Treat Rev 2003;29(6):533–40.
4. Nathoo N, Chahlavi A, Barnett GH, et al. Pathobiology of brain metastases. J Clin Pathol 2005; 58(3):237–42.
5. Bremnes RM, Veve R, Hirsch FR, et al. The E-cadherin cell-cell adhesion complex and lung cancer invasion, metastasis, and prognosis. Lung Cancer 2002;36(2):115–24.
6. Shabani HK, Kitange G, Tsunoda K, et al. Immunohistochemical expression of E-cadherin in metastatic brain tumors. Brain Tumor Pathol 2003;20(1): 7–12.
7. Yoshimasu T, Sakurai T, Oura S, et al. Increased expression of integrin alpha3beta1 in highly brain metastatic subclone of a human non-small cell lung cancer cell line. Cancer Sci 2004;95(2): 142–8.
8. Carbonell WS, Ansorge O, Sibson N, et al. The vascular basement membrane as "soil" in brain metastasis. PLoS One 2009;4(6):e5857.
9. Zheng Y, Lu Z. Paradoxical roles of FAK in tumor cell migration and metastasis. Cell Cycle 2009;8(21): 3474–9.
10. Zheng Y, Xia Y, Hawke D, et al. FAK phosphorylation by ERK primes ras-induced tyrosine dephosphorylation of FAK mediated by PIN1 and PTP-PEST. Mol Cell 2009;35(1):11–25.
11. Yamamoto M, Ueno Y, Hayashi S, et al. The role of proteolysis in tumor invasiveness in glioblastoma and metastatic brain tumors. Anticancer Res 2002; 22(6C):4265–8.
12. Vassalli JD, Sappino AP, Belin D. The plasminogen activator/plasmin system. J Clin Invest 1991;88(4): 1067–72.
13. Marchetti D, Denkins Y, Reiland J, et al. Brain-metastatic melanoma: a neurotrophic perspective. Pathol Oncol Res 2003;9(3):147–58.
14. Denkins Y, Reiland J, Roy M, et al. Brain metastases in melanoma: roles of neurotrophins. Neuro-oncol 2004;6(2):154–65.
15. Marchetti D, Nicolson GL. Human heparanase: a molecular determinant of brain metastasis. Adv Enzyme Regul 2001;41:343–59.
16. Bindal AK, Hammoud M, Shi WM, et al. Prognostic significance of proteolytic enzymes in human brain tumors. J Neurooncol 1994;22(2):101–10.
17. Stamenkovic I. Extracellular matrix remodelling: the role of matrix metalloproteinases. J Pathol 2003; 200(4):448–64.
18. Jaalinoja J, Herva R, Korpela M, et al. Matrix metalloproteinase 2 (MMP-2) immunoreactive protein is associated with poor grade and survival in brain neoplasms. J Neurooncol 2000;46(1):81–90.
19. Arnold SM, Young AB, Munn RK, et al. Expression of p53, bcl-2, E-cadherin, matrix metalloproteinase-9, and tissue inhibitor of metalloproteinases-1 in paired primary tumors and brain metastasis. Clin Cancer Res 1999;5(12):4028–33.

20. Kruger A, Sanchez-Sweatman OH, Martin DC, et al. Host TIMP-1 overexpression confers resistance to experimental brain metastasis of a fibrosarcoma cell line. Oncogene 1998;16(18):2419–23.

21. Khaitan D, Sankpal UT, Weksler B, et al. Role of KCNMA1 gene in breast cancer invasion and metastasis to brain. BMC Cancer 2009;9:258.

22. Verkman AS. Knock-out models reveal new aquaporin functions. Handb Exp Pharmacol 2009;190:359–81.

23. Lee JH, Welch DR. Suppression of metastasis in human breast carcinoma MDA-MB-435 cells after transfection with the metastasis suppressor gene, KiSS-1. Cancer Res 1997;57(12):2384–7.

24. Shirasaki F, Takata M, Hatta N, et al. Loss of expression of the metastasis suppressor gene KiSS1 during melanoma progression and its association with LOH of chromosome 6q16.3-q23. Cancer Res 2001;61(20):7422–5.

25. Dong JT, Suzuki H, Pin SS, et al. Down-regulation of the KAI1 metastasis suppressor gene during the progression of human prostatic cancer infrequently involves gene mutation or allelic loss. Cancer Res 1996;56(19):4387–90.

26. Yang X, Welch DR, Phillips KK, et al. A putative marker for metastatic potential in human breast cancer. Cancer Lett 1997;119(2):149–55.

27. Phillips KK, White AE, Hicks DJ, et al. Correlation between reduction of metastasis in the MDA-MB-435 model system and increased expression of the Kai-1 protein. Mol Carcinog 1998;21(2):111–20.

28. Takaoka A, Hinoda Y, Sato S, et al. Reduced invasive and metastatic potentials of KAI1-transfected melanoma cells. Jpn J Cancer Res 1998;89(4):397–404.

29. Shevde LA, Welch DR. Metastasis suppressor pathways—an evolving paradigm. Cancer Lett 2003;198(1):1–20.

30. Odintsova E, Sugiura T, Berditchevski F. Attenuation of EGF receptor signaling by a metastasis suppressor, the tetraspanin CD82/KAI-1. Curr Biol 2000;10(16):1009–12.

31. Guan RJ, Ford HL, Fu Y, et al. Drg-1 as a differentiation-related, putative metastatic suppressor gene in human colon cancer. Cancer Res 2000;60(3):749–55.

32. Shah MA, Kemeny N, Hummer A, et al. Drg1 expression in 131 colorectal liver metastases: correlation with clinical variables and patient outcomes. Clin Cancer Res 2005;11(9):3296–302.

33. Nam DH, Jeon HM, Kim S, et al. Activation of notch signaling in a xenograft model of brain metastasis. Clin Cancer Res 2008;14(13):4059–66.

34. Saito N, Hatori T, Murata N, et al. Comparison of metastatic brain tumour models using three different methods: the morphological role of the pia mater. Int J Exp Pathol 2008;89(1):38–44.

35. Huysentruyt LC, Mukherjee P, Banerjee D, et al. Metastatic cancer cells with macrophage properties: evidence from a new murine tumor model. Int J Cancer 2008;123(1):73–84.

36. Bos PD, Zhang XH, Nadal C, et al. Genes that mediate breast cancer metastasis to the brain. Nature 2009;459(7249):1005–9.

37. Salmaggi A, Maderna E, Calatozzolo C, et al. CXCL12, CXCR4 and CXCR7 expression in brain metastases. Cancer Biol Ther 2009;8(17):1608–14.

38. Martin B, Aragues R, Sanz R, et al. Biological pathways contributing to organ-specific phenotype of brain metastatic cells. J Proteome Res 2008;7(3):908–20.

39. Nguyen DX, Chiang AC, Zhang XH, et al. WNT/TCF signaling through LEF1 and HOXB9 mediates lung adenocarcinoma metastasis. Cell 2009;138(1):51–62.

40. Zhang C, Zhang F, Tsan R, et al. Transforming growth factor-beta2 is a molecular determinant for site-specific melanoma metastasis in the brain. Cancer Res 2009;69(3):828–35.

41. Braun S, Pantel K, Muller P, et al. Cytokeratin-positive cells in the bone marrow and survival of patients with stage I, II, or III breast cancer. N Engl J Med 2000;342(8):525–33.

42. Gao AC, Lou W, Sleeman JP, et al. Metastasis suppression by the standard CD44 isoform does not require the binding of prostate cancer cells to hyaluronate. Cancer Res 1998;58(11):2350–2.

43. Gao AC, Lou W, Dong JT, et al. CD44 is a metastasis suppressor gene for prostatic cancer located on human chromosome 11p13. Cancer Res 1997;57(5):846–9.

44. Lou W, Krill D, Dhir R, et al. Methylation of the CD44 metastasis suppressor gene in human prostate cancer. Cancer Res 1999;59(10):2329–31.

45. Harabin-Slowinska M, Slowinski J, Konecki J, et al. Expression of adhesion molecule CD44 in metastatic brain tumors. Folia Neuropathol 1998;36(3):179–84.

46. Li H, Liu J, Hofmann M, et al. Differential CD44 expression patterns in primary brain tumours and brain metastases. Br J Cancer 1995;72(1):160–3.

47. Li J, Yen C, Liaw D, et al. PTEN, a putative protein tyrosine phosphatase gene mutated in human brain, breast, and prostate cancer. Science 1997;275(5308):1943–7.

48. Tamura M, Gu J, Matsumoto K, et al. Inhibition of cell migration, spreading, and focal adhesions by tumor suppressor PTEN. Science 1998;280(5369):1614–7.

49. Tamura M, Gu J, Takino T, et al. Tumor suppressor PTEN inhibition of cell invasion, migration, and growth: differential involvement of focal adhesion kinase and p130Cas. Cancer Res 1999;59(2):442–9.

50. Hahn M, Wieland I, Koufaki ON, et al. Genetic alterations of the tumor suppressor gene PTEN/MMAC1 in human brain metastases. Clin Cancer Res 1999; 5(9):2431–7.

51. Chang C, Werb Z. The many faces of metalloproteases: cell growth, invasion, angiogenesis and metastasis. Trends Cell Biol 2001;11(11):S37–43.

52. Kim LS, Huang S, Lu W, et al. Vascular endothelial growth factor expression promotes the growth of breast cancer brain metastases in nude mice. Clin Exp Metastasis 2004;21(2):107–18.

53. Xia W, Unger P, Miller L, et al. The src-suppressed C kinase substrate, SSeCKS, is a potential metastasis inhibitor in prostate cancer. Cancer Res 2001; 61(14):5644–51.

54. Bergers G, Brekken R, McMahon G, et al. Matrix metalloproteinase-9 triggers the angiogenic switch during carcinogenesis. Nat Cell Biol 2000;2(10): 737–44.

55. Kono S, Rao JS, Bruner JM, et al. Immunohistochemical localization of plasminogen activator inhibitor type 1 in human brain tumors. J Neuropathol Exp Neurol 1994;53(3):256–62.

56. Roodink I, Verrijp K, Raats J, et al. Plexin D1 is ubiquitously expressed on tumor vessels and tumor cells in solid malignancies. BMC Cancer 2009;9:297.

57. Palmieri D, Fitzgerald D, Shreeve SM, et al. Analyses of resected human brain metastases of breast cancer reveal the association between upregulation of hexokinase 2 and poor prognosis. Mol Cancer Res 2009;7(9):1438–45.

58. Yaguchi H, Ohkura N, Tsukada T, et al. Menin, the multiple endocrine neoplasia type 1 gene product, exhibits GTP-hydrolyzing activity in the presence of the tumor metastasis suppressor nm23. J Biol Chem 2002;277(41):38197–204.

59. Ouatas T, Salerno M, Palmieri D, et al. Basic and translational advances in cancer metastasis: nm23. J Bioenerg Biomembr 2003;35(1):73–9.

60. Sarris M, Scolyer RA, Konopka M, et al. Cytoplasmic expression of nm23 predicts the potential for cerebral metastasis in patients with primary cutaneous melanoma. Melanoma Res 2004;14(1):23–7.

61. Seraj MJ, Samant RS, Verderame MF, et al. Functional evidence for a novel human breast carcinoma metastasis suppressor, BRMS1, encoded at chromosome 11q13. Cancer Res 2000;60(11):2764–9.

62. Seraj MJ, Harding MA, Gildea JJ, et al. The relationship of BRMS1 and RhoGDI2 gene expression to metastatic potential in lineage related human bladder cancer cell lines. Clin Exp Metastasis 2000;18(6):519–25.

63. Liu Y, El-Naggar S, Darling DS, et al. Zeb1 links epithelial-mesenchymal transition and cellular senescence. Development 2008;135(3):579–88.

64. Wrage M, Ruosaari S, Eijk PP, et al. Genomic profiles associated with early micrometastasis in lung cancer: relevance of 4q deletion. Clin Cancer Res 2009;15(5):1566–74.

65. Grinberg-Rashi H, Ofek E, Perelman M, et al. The expression of three genes in primary non-small cell lung cancer is associated with metastatic spread to the brain. Clin Cancer Res 2009;15(5):1755–61.

66. Narla G, DiFeo A, Fernandez Y, et al. KLF6-SV1 overexpression accelerates human and mouse prostate cancer progression and metastasis. J Clin Invest 2008;118(8):2711–21.

67. Micalizzi DS, Christensen KL, Jedlicka P, et al. The six1 homeoprotein induces human mammary carcinoma cells to undergo epithelial-mesenchymal transition and metastasis in mice through increasing TGF-beta signaling. J Clin Invest 2009;119(9): 2678–90.

Review of Imaging Techniques in the Diagnosis and Management of Brain Metastases

Angela Lignelli, MD[a],*, Alexander G. Khandji, MD[b]

KEYWORDS

- Brain metastasis • Imaging techniques
- Advanced imaging techniques • Metastatic disease

Brain metastasis is one of the most common diagnoses encountered by neurologists, neurosurgeons, radiologists, and oncologists. The aim of this article is to review imaging modalities used in the diagnosis and follow-up of brain metastases. Through the use of various imaging techniques more accurate preoperative diagnosis and more precise intraoperative planning can be made. Post-treatment evaluation can also be refined through the use of these imaging techniques.

Metastatic disease to the brain affects approximately 10% to 20% of cancer patients[1] but can be much higher depending on which data series is reviewed (radiologic, surgical, or autopsy). The overall incidence of metastatic brain disease is increasing, which has paralleled the rise in primary lung cancer. Another factor contributing to this increase is the longer survival rates in patients with metastases due to improvements in therapy and better radiologic detection.[2] With respect to autopsy and clinical data, which are more difficult to verify, the incidence of brain metastases is likely to be higher than that of primary brain tumors.[3–5]

The general location of metastases in the brain is consistent with blood flow, with approximately 80% in the cerebral hemispheres, 15% in the cerebellum, and 5% in the brain stem.[6,7] Brain metastases occur secondary to hematogenous spread of neoplastic cells to the brain or tumor emboli.[8] Metastases may also involve the calvarium, dura, and leptomeninges, but parenchymal metastases are the most common. The most common sources of metastases are lung (40% to 50%), breast (15% to 25%), and melanoma (5% to 20%).[9] Gastrointestinal and renal cell carcinomas are less common but not infrequent. Melanoma is the most likely neoplasm to metastasize to the brain (approximately 50%).[10,11] Although metastases may be multiple (eg, melanoma), solitary metastases are not uncommon, as seen in lung and breast cancers (approximately 50%).[5]

GENERAL IMAGING CHARACTERISTICS

There is no particular location predilection with regard to tumor origin, with a few exceptions. Renal cancer is seen slightly more commonly infratentorially (**Fig. 1**). This may be secondary to retrograde dissemination via Batson plexus, which may account for a slightly higher incidence of posterior fossa metastases from retroperitoneal tumors, such as those of the gastrointestinal tract, bladder, kidney, and uterus.[12–14]

A common general location of parenchymal metastases is the interface of cortical brain and white matter tracts (ie, the gray-white junction),

[a] Neuroradiology Division, Radiology Department, Columbia University, New York Presbyterian Medical Center, Milstein Hospital Room 3-101, 177 Fort Washington Avenue, New York, NY 10032, USA
[b] Neuroradiology Division, Radiology Department, Columbia University, New York Presbyterian Medical Center, New York, NY 10032, USA
* Corresponding author.
E-mail address: al270@columbia.edu

Neurosurg Clin N Am 22 (2011) 15–25
doi:10.1016/j.nec.2010.09.002
1042-3680/11/$ — see front matter © 2011 Elsevier Inc. All rights reserved.

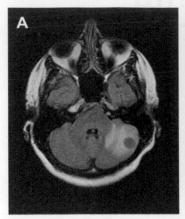
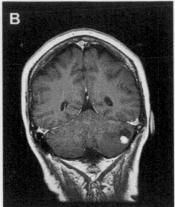

Fig. 1. Renal cell carcinoma solitary metastasis. (*A*) FLAIR sequence demonstrates a hypointense lesion with significant surrounding edema. (*B*) Cystic mass with associated nodule.

which may be accounted for by the significant change in size of arterioles from cortex to white matter, resulting in lodging of metastases in this location (**Fig. 2**).

In addition, metastases are usually surrounded by extensive vasogenic edema. This may be due to tumor capillaries' increased permeability with respect to normal capillaries as well as temporary occlusion as a result of neoplastic cell growth.[15,16] This abnormal vascular permeability allows macromolecules to travel easily into the perivascular and then interstitial spaces. These changes cause increase in pressure on the arterial side of capillary bed and increase in transudation.[17–19] As a result, peritumoral vasogenic edema, which follows white matter, interdigitating with uninvolved gray matter can be observed on CT but is more obvious on MRI. Cortical metastases, therefore, may not exhibit much surrounding edema because the cortex has a tight interstitium. These metastases may be missed without contrast on

both CT and MRI, due to their lack of reactive edema.[15]

Most metastases are hypodense on noncontrast CT but may not be well visualized amidst the surrounding hypodense edema. The pattern of MRI signal intensity of different metastases is not usually helpful in providing a specific diagnosis, but a few general observations have been made. Most metastases demonstrate prolonged relaxation time (high T2 signal).[20] Metastases may demonstrate cystic necrosis. Low T1 and high T2 signal, however, does not confirm the cystic nature of a neoplasm. Sharp demarcation of lesion with rim enhancement should also be observed. Unlike simple cysts, cystic necrosis demonstrates high signal on fluid-attenuated inversion recovery (FLAIR) sequence (which suppresses signal intensity that is cerebral spinal fluid [CSF]-like). Usually, the T1 rim is not high as expected with an abscess. Necrosis, however, can also shorten relaxation time (low T2 signal).[21] This may be secondary to

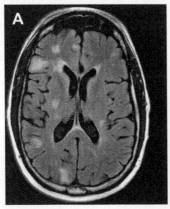
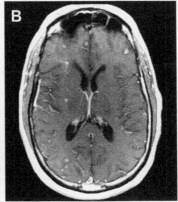

Fig. 2. Poorly differentiated adenocarcinoma lung metastases. (*A*) FLAIR sequence demonstrates multiple hyperintense lesions primarily involving the gray-white junction. (*B*) Postcontrast, these lesions demonstrate prominent enhancement.

paramagnetics within the tumor (eg, iron or copper) or free radical peroxidation.

Hemorrhage can be associated with metastatic neoplasm and is easily identified acutely on CT as hyperdensity, which decreases in attenuation after 3 to 4 days, becoming isodense and subsequently hypodense by approximately 7 to 10 days. The paramagnetic effects of blood breakdown products allow intratumoral hemorrhage to be readily identified on MRI for weeks to years after the acute event. Approximately 20% of metastases are hemorrhagic and a hemorrhagic neoplasm is more likely to be metastatic than primary. The most common hemorrhagic metastases are melanoma, small cell lung cancer, thyroid cancer, choriocarcinoma, and renal cell carcinoma **Fig. 3**.[22]

Hemorrhagic metastases, like other hemorrhagic neoplasms, may demonstrate heterogeneous intensity pattern (due to repeated bleeding), an incomplete hemosiderin rim,

disproportionate amount of edema for hematoma size, or persistent/increasing edema over several weeks. These findings suggest an underlying neoplasm. Additional characteristics that may help to distinguish an uncomplicated parenchymal hematoma from a hemorrhagic metastasis include delayed evolution of hemorrhage within the neoplasm (persistent deoxyhemoglobin-usually seen only for 3 to 5 days) and T1 shortening of intracellular methemoglobin within and not at the periphery of the lesion. Identification of enhancing, non-hemorrhagic tumor component can often seal the diagnosis of hemorrhagic metastasis.[23,24]

Melanin-containing melanoma metastasis also typically demonstrates T1 shortening (high signal on T1) and isointense T2 signal due to free radical content of melanin, unlike intracellular methemoglobin, which demonstrates high T1 and very low T2 signal. Confounding this observation is the occurrence of hemorrhage within melanoma metastases. With associated use of a susceptibility

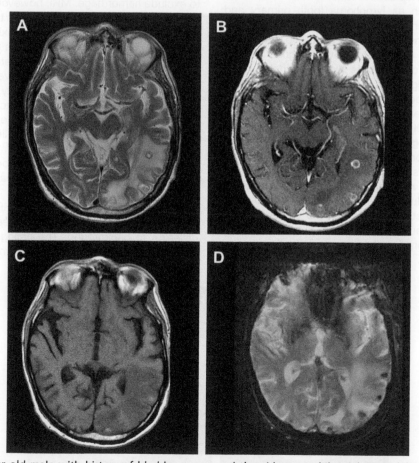

Fig. 3. 78 year old male with history of bladder cancer and thyroid cancer. (*A*) Axial T2 and (*B*) postcontrast T1-weighted sequence demonstrate several left temporal enhancing lesions. (*C*) Precontrast T1 sequence lesions demonstrate T1 shortening. (*D*) Lesions demonstrate low gradient recalled echo (GRE) signal compatible with hemorrhagic metastases.

sequence, T2*, further improved detection of melanoma metastases is possible. At times, melanoma lesions are detected only on T2*-weighted (also known as gradient-echo) sequence (**Fig. 4**). Amelanotic melanoma demonstrates T1 hypointensity and T2 hyperintensity.[25]

Hypervascularity can be associated with a metastatic lesion, with possible subsequent hemorrhage. Prominent flow voids seen on T2-weighted sequence represent enlarged vessels. The differential diagnosis includes hemangioblastoma, glioblastoma multiforme (GBM), anaplastic oligodendroglioma, and metastatic renal cell carcinoma. Gradient recalled echo (GRE) sequence can confirm both the presence of hemorrhage and prominent vessels.

Low T2 signal (similar to gray matter) is seen in some metastatic neoplasms and may offer a clue to tissue of origin. Mucin-secreting tumors (gastrointestinal and genitourinary adenocarcinomas and at times lung) and hypercellular neoplasms (high nuclear-to-cytoplasmic ratio, small round cell tumors), such as lymphoma (both primary and metastatic), medulloblastoma/primitive neuroectodermal tumors, pineoblastoma, and neuroblastomas, often demonstrate low T2 signal.[26] These lesions also demonstrate slightly restricted diffusion (high signal on diffusion weighted imaging [DWI] with corresponding reduced apparent diffusion coefficient [ADC] maps), again due to their high cellularity and decreased interstitial space and water **Fig. 5**.[15] Small cell lung cancer, amelanotic melanoma, and some hemorrhagic metastases may also have low T2 signal.

Calcified metastases are rare and most commonly due to ovarian cancer and osteosarcoma metastases. Calcifications are best seen on CT, because MRI may not provide sufficient discrimination between calcification and hemorrhage.[27]

CONTRAST-ENHANCED MRI AND CT

Contrast enhancement is necessary to evaluate for metastatic disease, because nearly all metastases demonstrate enhancement due to lack of blood-brain barrier and lack of blood-tumor barrier in their vascular endothelium. The pattern of enhancement can vary significantly among different metastatic neoplasms but again offers little clue as to the tissue origin. The enhancement pattern may be solid, peripheral, or nodular. The wall characteristics may help distinguish a neoplasm, either metastatic or primary, from a benign process, such as abscess or demyelinating disorder. Irregular thick or nodular enhancement is more commonly seen with malignant neoplasm than with benign conditions, which usually produce smooth thin wall enhancement.

MRI without and with contrast is the imaging modality of choice in evaluating patients with suspected metastases.[28] Head CT is often performed at the initial screening or in an emergency setting to exclude hemorrhage. MRI, however, is superior to CT either without or with contrast in the detection and evaluation of metastases. Approximately 19% of patients with a solitary metastasis on contrast-enhanced CT have multiple metastases on a contrast-enhanced MRI.[29] Improved detection with postcontrast MRI is secondary to superior soft tissue contrast, lack of bone artifact, decreased partial volume averaging, and better enhancement with paramagnetic MRI agents (gadolinium agents) versus CT iodinated contrasts.[28–30] In addition, MRI is better able to identify posterior fossa/infratentorial lesions and leptomeningeal metastatic disease.

Identification of lesions on MRI depends primarily on size of lesion and degree of contrast of lesion to background. The timing and dosing of imaging after gadolinium contrast

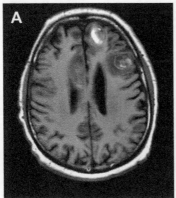 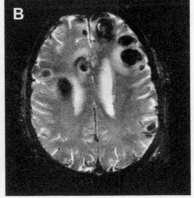

Fig. 4. Melanoma metastases. (*A*) T1 shortening. (*B*) GRE sequence demonstrates several additional lesions not seen on T1 sequence.

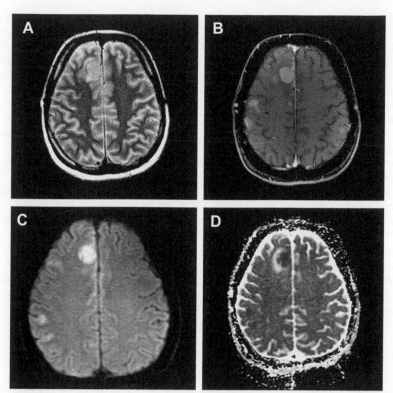

Fig. 5. Metastatic primitive neuroectodermal tumor in a 20-year-old man. (*A, B*) Isointense T2 signal in a solidly enhancing mass. (*C*) High DWI signal. (*D*) Corresponding low ADC map consistent with restricted diffusion.

administration play a major role in visualizing metastases. Delayed imaging postcontrast administration may help in detection of lesions that are 5 mm or smaller. Waiting 5 to 35 minutes with standard dose improves detection.[29,31,32] Higher dosing also detects more lesions and approximately 10% of such cases alter management. With triple dosing, Yuh and colleagues[33] found improved detection of multiple metastases. Delineation of these lesions may be important in developing a therapeutic strategy for a patient. Furthermore, prognostic factors after treatment vary depending on the number of cerebral metastases.[34]

Another option for improved visualization of smaller metastases is the use of higher-field MRI scanners. 3T MRI scanners, now readily available in clinical practice, have higher signal-to-noise ratio and longer T1 relaxation time of gray and white matter, which results in more shortening of T1 relaxation time by the uptake of contrast. Flow artifacts are more noticeable at higher field strengths and can mimic small metastases but can be readily reduced with saturation pulses.[35]

MR techniques, such as magnetization transfer with single-dose gadolinium diethylenetriamine penta-acetic acid (Gd-DTPA), have also been found as efficient as triple-dose Gd-DTPA. Magnetization transfer allows better visualization of intracranial lesions by preapplying an off-resonance radio frequency pulse, which suppresses the signal of the background tissue.[36] Knauth and colleagues[36] studied 24 patients with 34 enhancing intracranial lesions. No difference was found in number of lesions detected when comparing standard-dose magnetization transfer T1-weighted images with triple-dose T1-weighted images. Triple-dose magnetization transfer T1-weighted studies further increase lesion-to-white matter contrast but do not show additional lesions.

Use of magnetization transfer technique and higher-field magnet scanners, rather than triple dosing, should be considered, particularly in the setting of patients with renal disease, given recent concerns for nephrogenic systemic fibrosis or nephrogenic fibrosing dermopathy, which has been seen in patients with moderate to severe end-stage renal disease after the administration of a high dose of a gadolinium-based contrast agent.

DWI

DWI is commonly used in MRI brain studies. DWI reflects the microscopic motion of water in tissue is usually disorganized or Brownian motion. DWI depends primarily on water motion in the extracellular space, with increased signal seen when it is not moving freely. To quantify the degree of water motion, ADC maps are needed, which depict true restriction as dark. The more restricted the motion of water, the lower the ADC value, with darker ADC maps. Conventional DWI imaging is commonly used in the setting of acute stroke where decreased diffusion is present, thought to be secondary to cytotoxic edema and decreased extracellular space.[37,38]

Necrotic neoplasms can be differentiated from bacterial abscess using DWI and ADC maps. Bacterial abscesses tend to demonstrate increased DWI signal and corresponding decreased ADC values. This reduced diffusion may be due to decreased movement of water molecules by bacteria, inflammatory cells, cellular debris, and macromolecules, such as fibrinogen, found in viscous purulent fluid.[39] In addition, bacterial abscesses tend to demonstrate a complete or partial, markedly hypointense T2 rim.[40] This finding, together with restricted diffusion, can accurately discriminate cystic or necrotic neoplasm from brain abscess (**Fig. 6**). In partly treated abscesses, however, restricted diffusion may not be observed.

Typically, metastatic neoplasms exhibit an elevated ADC, but there is significant overlap with the ADC values of primary neoplasms. In some studiers, necrotic metastases demonstrated some restricted diffusion, as expected with a bacterial abscess.[41–43] Attempts have been made to correlate DWI signal intensity with tumor histology in solid neoplasms. Higher mean ADC values with DWI hypointensity were observed in well differentiated versus poorly differentiated adenocarcinomas (with low signal on T2) and metastases other than adenocarcinoma.[44] Small cell carcinoma has also shown hyperintensity on DWI, with low ADC values.[44,45]

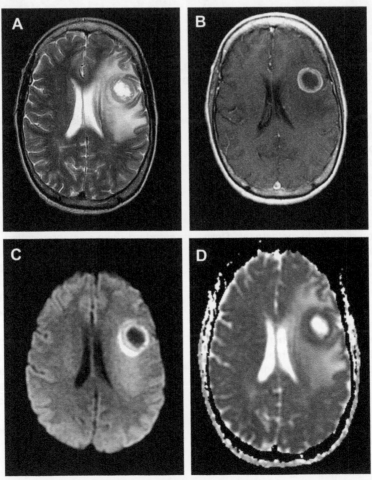

Fig. 6. Lung adenocarcinoma solitary metastasis. (*A, B*) Cystic mass with severe surrounding edema. (*C, D*) DWI signal is low with high ADC compatible with neoplasm.

It is the ADC value in the peritumoral edema that may offer a clue as to the diagnosis of an unknown lesion. Chiang and coworkers[46] found that the ADC values of peritumoral edema of metastases and contrast-enhancing areas significantly higher than those in high-grade gliomas. This may be due to higher intra- and extracellular water fractions in metastases than in high-grade gliomas. In addition, the significant increase in ADC in edema surrounding metastases may be due to more fluid production. Primary gliomas, alternatively, have infiltrating cells in the surrounding edema and ADC values might show areas of infiltration.[46]

An extension of DWI is diffusion tensor imaging (DTI), which allows the measurement of direction as well as magnitude of water diffusion in 3-D space. MRI diffusion tensors are generated by applying diffusion gradients symmetrically in at least six radial directions (typically 20 or more). From these, a tensor matrix is converted into differential equations, which yield an eigenvector, reflecting magnitude and direction of diffusion in 3-D space. Mean diffusivity (MD) can be calculated from the eigenvector (magnitude measure) and directionality can be quantified by using fractional anisotropy (FA). FA values range between 0, perfectly isotropic (spherical), and 1, linear.

Lower FA values are seen in edema or CSF where diffusion is more spherical and higher FA values are seen in normal white matter tracts where water diffusion is highly directional. The FA value is used in DTI tractography to define the threshold for accepting a voxel as representative of a white matter tract (eg, FA >0.20). A pitfall to remember when interpreting DTI tractography images is that although low FA in white matter may indicate altered diffusion with axon disruption or dysfunction, the presence of edema around otherwise intact axons can produce the false appearance of interrupted or damaged white matter tracts.

DTI is used in preoperative planning to identify white matter tracts that need to be preserved during surgery while maximizing resection margins. Yu and colleagues[47] studied 16 patients with brain tumors, both primary and metastatic, and found that diffusion tensor tractography was beneficial in the neurosurgical planning and postoperative assessment.

On conventional MRI, solitary metastases and high-grade gliomas often exhibit similar signal and contrast patterns. In general, both classes of neoplasm exhibit significant surrounding high T2 signal, or vasogenic edema. Lu and colleagues[48] performed DTI on 12 patients with high-grade gliomas and 12 with metastatic lesions. With respect to normal white matter, statistically significant changes are seen in the MD and FA values of the peritumoral T2 signal abnormalities. High-grade neoplasms, however, could not be differentiated from metastatic lesions using peritumoral FA changes, but the peritumoral MD surrounding metastatic lesions was found significantly greater than that surrounding gliomas.[48] MD is likely related to increases in extracellular water, which is greater in vasogenic edema surrounding metastasis.[8] In addition, both increased water content and tumor infiltration can cause more disorganized diffusion and, therefore, decreased FA. So, FA peritumoral changes are similar in high grade gliomas and metastasis—increased water content and tumor cells in high-grade gliomas is equivalent to increased water content alone in metastases.[49,50]

MAGNETIC RESONANCE PERFUSION

Perfusion studies were initially performed using nuclear medicine techniques with positron emission tomography (PET) and single-photon emission CT (SPECT) scanners using radioactive tracers. SPECT studies are commonly performed using 99mTc-hexamethylpropylene amine oxime (99mTc-HMPAO) whereas PET studies for perfusion use Oxygen-15-water (O-15 H_2O). Magnetic resonance (MR) perfusion studies are commonly performed using dynamic susceptibility contrast technique or bolus tracking. A more recent MR perfusion method is arterial spin labeling, which does not require contrast administration. Spins in the inflow arteries are perturbed with radiofrequency pulses and the effect of these perturbed spins on image intensity after they flow into the slice is measured.

Although contrast enhancement demonstrates a breakdown in the blood-brain barrier, it is not measuring underlying local neovascularity. Regional cerebral blood volume maps (rCBV) calculated from perfusion studies have been used to determine microvasculature. A statistically significant correlation has been found between rCBV and glioma grade, with high-grade gliomas demonstrating higher rCBV.[51–53]

Several recent studies have addressed the use of perfusion imaging in differentiating between high-grade gliomas and metastases. The rCBV values within the high-grade gliomas versus metastases are not significantly different.[51,54] The peritumoral edema of primary high-grade glioma has peritumoral infiltrating cells whereas the peritumoral edema of metastatic lesions does not.

Law and colleagues, in 2002,[55] and Chiang and colleagues, in 2004,[46] in 2004, noted that rCBV in the peritumoral region is significantly higher in primary gliomas than metastases.[54] The peritumoral area surrounding metastases that demonstrates high T2 signal is likely due to vasogenic edema associated with abnormal capillaries of tissue of origin that have increase leakiness.[8] In addition, blood flow in edematous tissue is decreased secondary to local compression of microcirculation by the extravasated fluid.[49] In high-grade gliomas, there is breakdown of the blood-blain barrier in the enhancing component. In the peritumoral region, however, the hyperintense T2 signal likely reflects both vasogenic edema and tumor infiltration, accounting for higher rCBV.[46,51,54]

MR SPECTROSCOPY

MR spectroscopy (MRS) allows the noninvasive evaluation of the chemical makeup of the brain. Proton spectroscopy is what is used in clinical practice. Single-voxel (where a single volume of tissue is excited) or multivoxel techniques are used for in vivo MRS. The proton spectra produced demonstrate peaks at specific resonant frequencies. Many compounds can be detected but several are more commonly used in clinical practice. Choline is a measure of membrane turnover, because it is involved in membrane synthesis and degradation (resonates at 3.2 ppm). Choline is usually increased with disorders that cause increase in cellular membrane turnover and in disease states that are associated with a hypercellularity. Creatine is a measure of cellular energy (involved in ATP generation and energy metabolism) and relatively constant in the brain, so it is used as a reference (3.02 ppm). N-acetylaspartate (NAA) is a marker of neuronal viability (both concentration and integrity). NAA is found in mature neurons and neuronal processes (resonates at 2.02 ppm) and is reduced in disorders that destroy or replace neurons. Lactic acid (1.33 ppm) measures anaerobic metabolism. It is an end product in glycolysis, which builds up when oxidative metabolism is unable to meet energy requirements and is normally very low. Lactic acid is elevated in acute stroke, recent seizure, and high-grade/necrotic neoplasms. Highly cellular lesions that outgrow their blood supply use up oxygen and rely on aneorobic glycolysis, with production of lactate. In addition, certain neoplasms have elevated glycolysis independent of oxidative metabolism. Myo-inositol is a cyclic sugar needed for cell growth and glucose storage. It has a prominent peak at 3.56 ppm that is mainly detected with a short echo time. Located in glia (astrocytes), it indicates gliosis if elevated and is usually decreased in high-grade primary brain neoplasms.[15] Lipid is seen in cellular breakdown (0.8 and 1.5 ppm) and is a marker of necrosis, as expected in high-grade malignancy both primary brain tumors and metastases.[15(pp112,111)] The general, nonspecific pattern for neoplasm is low NAA with high choline. In addition, lactate may be seen as neoplasms disrupt the normal glucose metabolism, with resulting hypoxia. Lipids may also be present in high grade neoplasms, secondary to necrosis. Regions with high lactate also have corresponding elevated CBV on perfusion studies. Elevated CBV is an indirect measure of angiogenesis- one of the features of malignant tumors. In general, ratios of these metabolites are used, such as NAA/Cr or Ch/NAA, and comparison is made of normal brain versus diseased brain. Absolute quantification of brain metabolites is not easy to calculate.[15]

Mishra and colleagues[56] used MRS and DWI in 52 patients to distinguish ring-enhancing cystic lesions: abscess versus nonabscess. Criteria of for abscess diagnosis of low ADC and presence of lactate and cytosolic amino acids (at 0.9 ppm) were observed in 25 of 29 cases of abscesses. Criteria for tumor cyst were hypointensity on DWI with higher ADC values and presence of lactate and choline, whereas for benign cyst the criteria were hypointensity on DWI with ADC equal to CSF and presence of lactate and choline as well as amino acids, succinate, and alanine. The sensitivity of DWI for differentiating brain abscess from nonbrain abscess was 72% and for spectroscopy 96%, with a reported specificity of 100% for both techniques.

Intratumoral spectral patterns may not be helpful in differentiating primary gliomas from metastases due to significant overlap.[57] The MR spectra of high-grade glioma compared with brain metastases demonstrate a similar pattern. Two comparative studies performed by the same research group using a long and short echo time 1H–MR signal evaluated differentiation of metastases and high-grade astrocytoma. The area under the receiver operating characteristic curve for differentiating these two groups of tumor was poor—64% and 59%, respectively. For all other comparisons, for example, GBM versus grade II astrocytomas and metastases versus astrocytoma grade II, the area under the receiver operating characteristic curve was 0.9.[58–60] A study by Law,[55] however, using a smaller group of patients, did find that the choline/creatine (Cho/Cr) ratio was significantly higher in GBM versus metastases. Opstad and colleagues[61] recently found a significant difference in lipid to macromolecules peaks, using a short echo time, between these two groups, with higher values for metastases. In an earlier study, Ishimaru and coworkers showed that creatine absence might indicate metastases whereas absence of lipid signal may exclude metastases.[62]

More consistent than intratumoral MRS is the finding that peritumoral Cho/Cr ratio can help differentiate between high-grade gliomas and metastases.[55] Elevated peritumoral Ch/Cr ratio was observed in high-grade gliomas but not in metastases. Again this is likely due to peritumoral infiltrating high-grade glioma cells.[46,55] No significant difference was observed for NAA/Cr in peritumoral areas, because there is no neuronal replacement or destruction in either metastases or high-grade glioma.[46]

FLUDEOXYGLUCOSE F 18

Fludeoxyglucose F 18 (^{18}F-FDG) PET has been used in the evaluation of lesions to determine their metabolic activity and has been used in brain tumor imaging. ^{18}F-FDG is actively transported across the blood-brain barrier and into the cell where it is phosphorylated. ^{18}F-FDG uptake is generally high in high-grade tumors.

DiChiro and colleagues,[63] in one of the first articles on PET, demonstrated that in all 10 patients with high-grade astrocytomas PET showed a region of high activity and a visible hot spot. This finding was not observed in any of the 13 patients with low-grade gliomas. Not all cases in this study, however, were biopsy proved. Many tumors have high glucose uptake and there is a correlation between uptake and anaplastic transformation. De Witte and colleagues[64] showed that the presence of areas of increased FDG uptake in a histologically proved low-grade tumor predicts, in most cases, a deleterious evolution to malignant transformation. Others have reported varying degrees of accuracy of PET in differentiating high-grade from low-grade tumors and high-grade tumors from radiation necrosis.

These conflicting reports are due to several limitations of brain PET imaging. Normal brain tissue has a high rate of glucose metabolism. When using PET to image low-grade tumors and even in some high-grade tumors, there may not be sufficient visual difference between normal and tumor glucose uptake to be detectable.[65] ^{18}F-FDG uptake in neoplasms can vary greatly; high-grade tumors may have uptake that is only similar to or slightly above that in white matter, especially after treatment.[66] In distinguishing radiation necrosis from recurrent brain rumors, 18F-FDG PET has provided mixed results depending on methods of analysis. If MRI structural information is available for correlation, however, significant improvement in sensitivity and specificity is noted. In a series of 44 lesions treated with stereotactic radiosurgery, 18F-FDG PET alone had a sensitivity of 65% in subjects with metastases but reached 86% when MRI and PET images were coregistered.[67]

In a retrospective study by Kosaka and colleagues,[68] FDG PET was evaluated in the differentiation of CNS lymphoma versus high-grade glioma versus metastatic brain tumor, in 34 patients. By using a standardized uptake value maximum, a cutoff level was obtained to distinguish lymphoma from high-grade gliomas and metastatic brain tumors. When comparing high-grade gliomas to metastatic brain tumors, gliomas tended to have higher standardized uptake values, but significant overlap was found.[68]

Whole-body PET can also be used in suspected brain metastasis to evaluate for the primary lesion.[69]

SUMMARY

Metastatic lesions can generally be evaluated with routine contrast MRI studies. Higher dosing of contrast agents, magnetization transfer technique, and higher field strength magnets increase sensitivity.

Typical characteristics of metastases, including multiplicity, location, and signal characteristics, together with clinical history, are often sufficient to suggest the diagnosis of metastatic intracranial disease. In the setting of more complex cases or solitary brain metastases, advanced MRI techniques and PET will aid in reaching a diagnosis.

ACKNOWLEDGMENTS

Special thanks to Dr Mark Stoopler, Dr Pallavi Utukuri and Dr David Chung for providing several of the images used in this manuscript.

REFERENCES

1. Barnholtz-Sloan JS, Sloan AE, Davis FG, et al. Incidence proportions of brain metastases in patients diagnosed (1973 to 2001) in the Metropolitan Detroit Cancer Surveillance System. J Clin Oncol 2004;22: 2865–72.
2. Johnson JD, Young B. Demographics of brain metastases. Neurosurg Clin N Am 1996;7:337.
3. Gavrilovic Igor T, Posner J. In 45% of surgical cases symptoms from brain metastases were experienced prior to a known diagnosis of primary cancer—atlas 260. J Neurooncol 2005;75:5–14.
4. Posner JB. Brain metastases: 1995. A brief review. J Neurooncol 1996;27:287–93.
5. Nussbaum ES, Djalilian HR, Cho KH, et al. Brain metastases. Histology, multiplicity, surgery, and survival. Cancer 1996;78:1781–8.

6. Delattre JY, Krol G, Thaler HT, et al. Distribution of brain metastases. Arch Neurol 1988;45:741–4.

7. Ewing J. Metastasis. In: Ewing J, editor. Neoplastic diseases: a treastise on tumours. Philadelphia: Saunders; 1940. p. 62–74.

8. Zhang M, Olsson Y. Hematogenous metastases of the human brain—characteristics of peritumoral brain changes: a review. J Neurooncol 1997;35(1): 81–9 [review].

9. Eichler A, Plotkin S. Brain metastases. Curr Treat Options Neurol 2008;10:308–14.

10. Amer MH, Al-Sarraf M, Baker LH, et al. Malignant melanoma and central nervous system metastases: incidence, diagnosis, treatment and survival. Cancer 1978;42:660–8.

11. O'Neill BP, Buckner JC, Coffey RJ, et al. Brain metastatic lesions. Mayo Clin Proc 1994;69:1062–8.

12. Hojo S, Hirano A. Pathology of metastases affecting the central nervous system. In: Takakura K, Sano K, Hojo S, et al, editors. Metastastic tumors of the central nervous system. Tokyo: Igaku-Shoin; 1982. p. 5.

13. Posner JB. Diagnosis and treatment of metastases to the brain. Clin Bull 1974;4:47.

14. Trillet V, Catajar JF, Croisile B, et al. Cerebral Metastases as first symptom of bronchogenic carcinoma. A prospective study of 37 cases. Cancer 1991;67: 2935.

15. Atlas S. Magnetic resonance imaging of the brain and spine, vol. 1 and 2. 4th edition. Lippincott Williams and Wilkins; 2009. p. 531–7, 1844–5.

16. Zimmerman HM. The pathology of primary brain tumors. Semin Roentgenol 1984;19:129–38.

17. Steen RG. Edema and tumor perfusion: characterization by quantitative 1H MR imaging. Am J Roentgenol 1992;158:259–64.

18. Sevick EM, Jam AK. Measurement of capillary filtration coefficient in a solid tumor. Cancer Res 1991;51: 1352–5.

19. Kuroiwa T, Shibutani M, Tajima T, et al. Hydrostatic pressure versus osmotic pressure in the development of vasogenic brain edema induced by cold injury. Adv Neurol 1990;52:11–9.

20. Komiyama M, Yagura H, Baba M, et al. MR imaging: possibility of tissue characterization of brain tumors using T1 and T2 values. AJNR Am J Neuroradiol 1987;8(1):65–70.

21. Kovalikova Z. Age-dependent variation of T1 and T2 relaxation times of adenocarcinoma in mice. Radiology 1987;164(2):543–8.

22. Mandybur TI. Intracranial hemorrhage caused by metastatic tumors. Neurology 1977;27(7):650–5.

23. Atlas SW, Grossman RI, Gomori JM, et al. Hemorrhagic intracranial malignant neoplasms:spin- echo MR imaging. Radiology 1987;164:71–7.

24. Destian S, Sze G, Krol G, et al. MR imaging of hemorrhagic intracranial neoplasms. AJR Am J Roentgenol 1989;152(1):137–44.

25. Gaviani P, Mullins M, Braga TA, et al. Improved Detection of metastatic melanoma by T2*-weighted imaging. AJNR Am J Neuroradiol 2006;27:605–8.

26. Carrier DA, Mawad ME, Kirkpatrick JB, et al. Metastatic adenocarcinoma to the brain: MR with pathologic correlation. AJNR Am J Neuroradiol 1994;15(1):155–9.

27. Hettmer S, Fleischhack G, Hasan C, et al. Intracranial manifestations of osteosarcoma. Pediatr Hematol Oncol 2002;19:347–54.

28. Healy ME, Hesselink JR, Press GA, et al. Increased detection of intracranial metastases with intravenous Gd-DTPA. Radiology 1987;165:619–24.

29. Schellinger PD, Meinck HM, Thron A. Diagnostic accuracy of MRI compared to CCT in patients with brain metastases. J Neurooncol 1999;44:275–81.

30. Davis PC, Hudgins PA, Peterman SB, et al. Diagnosis of cerebral metastases: double-dose delayed CT vs contrast-enhanced MR imaging. AJNR Am J Neuroradiol 1991;12(2):293–300.

31. Russell EJ, Geremia GK, Johnson CE, et al. Multiple cerebral metastases: detectability with Gd-DTPA-enhanced MR imaging. Radiology 1987;165:609–17.

32. Yuh WT, Tali ET, Nguyen HD, et al. The effect of contrast dose, imaging time, and lesion size in the MR detection of intracerebral metastasis. AJNR Am J Neuroradiol 1995;16(2):373–80.

33. Yuh WT, Fisher DJ, Runge VM, et al. Phase III multicenter trial of high-dose gadoteridol in MR evaluation of brain metastases. AJNR Am J Neuroradiol 1994;15(6):1037–51.

34. DiLuna ML, King JT Jr, Knisely JP, et al. Prognostic factors for survival after stereotactic radiosurgery vary with the number of cerebral metastases. Cancer 2007;109(1):135–45.

35. Trattnig S, Pinker K, Ba-Ssalamah A, et al. The optimal use of contrast agents at high field MRI. Eur Radiol 2006;16(6):1280–7. [Epub 2006 Mar 1].

36. Knauth M, Forsting M, Hartmann M. MR enhancement of brain lesions: increased contrast dose compared with magnetization transfer. AJNR Am J Neuroradiol 1996;17(10):1853–9.

37. Benveniste H, Hedlund LW, Johnson GA. Mechanism of detection of acute cerebral ischemia in rats by diffusion-weighted magnetic resonance microscopy. Stroke 1992;23(5):746–54.

38. Krabbe K, Gideon P, Wagn P, et al. MR diffusion imaging of human intracranial tumours. Neuroradiology 1997;39:483–9.

39. Ebisu T, Tanaka C, Umeda M, et al. Discrimination of brain abscess from necrotic or cystic tumors by diffusion weighted echo planar imaging. Magn Reson Imaging 1996;14:1113–6.

40. Fertikh D, Krejza J, Cunqueiro A, et al. Discrimination of capsular stage brain abscesses from necrotic or cystic neoplasms using diffusion-weighted magnetic resonance imaging. J Neurosurg 2007; 106(1):76–81.

41. Dorenbeck U, Butz B, Schlaier J, et al. Diffusion-weighted echo-planar MRI of the brain with calculated ADCs: a useful tool in the differential diagnosis of tumor necrosis from abscess? J Neuroimaging 2003;13(4):330−8.

42. Castillo M, Mukherji SK. Diffusion-weighted imaging in the evaluation of intracranial lesions. Semin Ultrasound CT MR 2000;21(6):405−16. Advanced MR Imaging Techniques.

43. Leuthardt EC, Wippold FJ 2nd, Oswood MC, et al. Diffusion-weighted MR imaging in the preoperative assessment of brain abscesses. Surg Neurol 2002; 58(6):395−402 [discussion: 402].

44. Hayashida Y, Hirai T, Morishita S, et al. Diffusion-weighted imaging of metastatic brain tumors: comparison with histologic type and tumor cellularity. AJNR Am J Neuroradiol 2006;27(7):1419−25.

45. Geijer B, Holtås S. Diffusion-weighted imaging of brain metastases: their potential to be misinterpreted as focal ischaemic lesions. Neuroradiology 2002;44(7):568−73. [Epub 2002 May 29].

46. Chiang IC, Kuo YT, Lu CY, et al. Distinction between high-grade gliomas and solitary metastases using peritumoral 3-T magnetic resonance spectroscopy, diffusion, and perfusion imagings. Neuroradiology 2004;46:619−27.

47. Yu CS, Li KC, Xuan Y, et al. Diffusion tensor tractography in patients with cerebral tumors: a helpful technique for neurosurgical planning and postoperative assessment. Eur J Radiol 2005;56(2):197−204.

48. Lu S, Ahn D, Johnson G, et al. Peritumoral diffusion tensor imaging of high-grade gliomas and metastatic brain tumors. AJNR Am J Neuroradiol 2003; 24(5):937−41.

49. Hossman KA, Bloink M. Blood flow and regulation of blood flow in experimental peritumoral edema. Stroke 1981;12:211−21.

50. Nabavi A, Black PM, Gering DT, et al. Serial intraoperative magnetic resonance imaging of brain shift. Neurosurgery 2001;48(4):787−97 [discussion: 797−8].

51. Rollin N, Guyotat J, Streichenberger N, et al. Clinical relevance of diffusion and perfusion magnetic resonance imaging in assessing intra-axial brain tumors. Neuroradiology 2006;48:150−9.

52. Knopp EA, Cha S, Johnson G, et al. Glial neoplasms: dynamic contrast-enhanced T2*-weighted MR imaging. Radiology 1999;211:791−8.

53. Shin JH, Lee HK, Kwun BD, et al. Using relative cerebral blood flow and volume to evaluate the histopathologic grade of cerebral gliomas: preliminary results. AJR Am J Roentgenol 2002;179(3):783−9.

54. Hakyemez B, Erdogan C, Gokalp G, et al. Solitary metastases and high-grade gliomas: radiological differentiation by morphometric analysis and perfusion-weighted MRI. Clin Radiol 2010;65(1):15−20.

55. Law M, Cha S, Knopp EA, et al. High-grade gliomas and solitary metastases: differentiation by using perfusion and proton spectroscopic MR imaging. Radiology 2002;222(3):715−21.

56. Mishra AM, Gupta RK, Jaggi RS, et al. Role of diffusion-weighted imaging and in vivo proton magnetic resonance spectroscopy in the differential diagnosis of ring-enhancing intracranial cystic mass lesions. J Comput Assist Tomogr 2004; 28(4):540−7.

57. Poptani H, Gupta RK, Roy R, et al. Characterization of intracranial mass lesions with in vivo protonMR spectroscopy. AJNR Am J Neuroradiol 1995;16: 1593−603.

58. Devos A, Lukas L, Suykens JA, et al. Classification of brain tumours using short echo time 1H MR spectra. J Magn Reson 2004;170(1):164−75.

59. Lukas L, Devos A, Suykens JA, et al. Brain tumour classification based on long echo time proton MRS signals. Artif Intell Med 2004;31:73−89.

60. Hollingworth W, Medina LS, Lenkinski RE, et al. A systematic literature review of magnetic resonance spectroscopy for the characterization of brain tumors. AJNR Am J Neuroradiol 2006;27(7):1404−11.

61. Opstad KS, Griffiths JR, Bell BA, et al. In vivo lipid T2 relaxation time measurements in high-grade tumors: differentiation of glioblastomas and metastases. In: Proceedings of the 11th Scientific Meeting and Exhibition (ISMRM 03). Toronto (Canada), July 10−16, 2003. p. 754.

62. Ishimaru H, Morikawa M, Iwanaga S, et al. Differentiation between high-grade glioma and metastatic brain tumor using single-voxel proton MR spectroscopy. Eur Radiol 2001;11(9):1784−91.

63. DiChiro G, DeLaPaz RL, Brooks RA, et al. Glucose utii- lization of cerebral gliomas measured by [¹IF] fluorodeoxyglucoseand positron emission tomography. Neurology 1982;32:1323−9.

64. De Witte O, Levivier M, Violon P, et al. Prognostic value of positron emission tomography with [18F] fluoro-2-D-glucose in the low-grade glioma. J Neurosurg 1996;39:470−7.

65. Chen W. Clinical applications of PET in brain tumors. J Nucl Med 2007;48(9):1468−81. [Epub 2007 Aug 17].

66. Wong TZ, van der Westhuizen GJ, Coleman RE. Positron emission tomography imaging of brain tumors. Neuroimaging Clin N Am 2002;12:615−26.

67. Chao ST, Suh JH, Raja S, et al. The sensitivity and specificity of FDG PET in distinguishing recurrent brain tumor from radionecrosis in patients treated with stereotactic radiosurgery. Int J Cancer 2001; 96(3):191−7.

68. Kosaka N, Tsuchida T, Uematsu H, et al. 18 FDG PET of common enhancing malignant brain tumors. AJR Am J Roentgenol 2008;190:W365−9.

69. Jeong HJ, Chung JK, Kim YK, et al. Usefulness of whole body (18) F-FDG PET in patients with suspected metastatic brain tumors. J Nucl Med 2002; 43:1432−7.

Medical Management of Brain Metastases

Nicholas Butowski, MD

KEYWORDS

- Adult • Brain metastases • Chemotherapy
- Medical oncology

Metastases to the brain are 5 to 10 times more common than primary brain tumors and commonly originate from the lung, breast, skin, kidney, and colon.[1] According to the 2008 American Cancer Society Registry, roughly 1.5 million Americans are diagnosed with cancer every year, and up to 40% of these patients, over a half million people annually, will develop one or more brain metastases.[2] Brain metastases may be identified in asymptomatic patients or present as headaches, seizures, mental status changes, and motor or sensory deficits. Additionally, the incidence of brain metastasis appears to be increasing likely due to the number of systemic cancer patients living long enough to develop metastases as a result of improved primary cancer therapies.[3] Treatment for patients with brain metastases should be individualized and balanced with regard to patient-specific and cancer-specific characteristics.[4] The main objective of treating brain metastases is to improve survival and to reduce symptom burden, preserve function, and enhance quality of life. As such, concurrent local control of existing brain metastases, prevention of future metastasis elsewhere in the brain, and control of the systemic cancer are required. The treatment modalities used to achieve these aims, either alone or in combination, include surgery, radiation, and medical therapy. This article is devoted to the medical management of brain metastases, namely the role of medical treatments and chemotherapy. Radiation therapy and surgery are discussed in detail elsewhere; however, a brief discussion of all of these modalities is included for the sake of thoroughness, and further information is available in several recent review articles.[1,3,5–9]

PATIENT PROGNOSTIC FACTORS

Prognostic factors maximize therapy for a patient and help avoid unnecessary and harmful treatment. The prognosis of patients with symptomatic brain metastases is poor, with a median survival in untreated patients of 4 weeks. Supportive care with corticosteroids increases survival to about 8 weeks, while more recognized treatments, like radiotherapy, lengthen the median survival time to roughly 4 months.[10] Several studies have attempted to identify factors that predict better survival.[11] In 1999, Lagerwaard and colleagues[12] published a retrospective review of 1292 patients with metastatic brain disease and identified prognostic factors. Eighty-four percent of the patients reviewed were treated with whole-brain radiation therapy (WBRT). Nine percent were treated with steroids only, and 7% were treated with surgery and radiotherapy. Data acquired included age, gender, Karnofsky performance status (KPS), number and distribution of brain metastases, site of primary tumor, histology, interval between primary tumor and brain metastases, systemic tumor activity, response to steroid treatment, and treatment modality. The overall median survival was 3.4 months, with 6-month, 1-year, and 2-year survival percentages of 36%, 12%, and 4%, respectively. Median survival was 1.3 months in patients treated with steroids alone, 3.6 months in patients treated with radiotherapy, and 8.9 months in patients treated with surgical resection followed by radiation. Multivariate analysis revealed that treatment modality was the most significant factor in predicting survival. Response to steroid treatment, performance status, systemic

The author has nothing to disclose.
Department of Neurological Surgery, University of California, 400 Parnassus Avenue # 0372, San Francisco, CA 94143, USA
E-mail address: Butowski@neurosurg.ucsf.edu

Neurosurg Clin N Am 22 (2011) 27–36
doi:10.1016/j.nec.2010.08.004
1042-3680/11/$ — see front matter
© 2011 Elsevier Inc. All rights reserved.

tumor activity, age, and number of metastases were also independent prognostic factors on survival, but secondary to treatment modality in level of significance.

More recent studies have confirmed these findings on prognostic factors.[13–15] Further analysis of the factors influencing the survival of patients with brain metastases resulted in the development of prognostic indexes.[14] The Recursive Partitioning Analysis (RPA), developed by the Radiation Therapy Oncology Group (RTOG), categorized patients who received WBRT into one of three prognostic groups. RPA class 1 represented patients younger than 65 years with a KPS of at least 70 and a controlled primary tumor with the brain the only site of metastases, resulting in a median survival of 7.1 months. RPA class 3 represented patients with a KPS less than 70, resulting in a median survival of 2.3 months. RPA class 2 represented all other patients, resulting in a median survival of 4.5 months.[16] The RPA, however, is limited by its subjective estimation of systemic tumor control and total brain metastases, two factors that influence survival.[17] Such factors are incorporated into the more recent Graded Prognostic Assessment (GPA), which has four factors (age, KPS, number of brain metastases, and the status of disease outside the central nervous system [CNS]) that partition patients into one of four categories, with median overall survival ranging from 2.6 to 11 months.[18] An even more recent study attempted to identify significant diagnosis-specific prognostic factors (Diagnosis-Specific Graded Prognostic Assessment [DS-GPA]).[7] This was done by retrospective analysis of 4259 patients with newly diagnosed brain metastases using univariate and multivariate analyses of the prognostic factors and outcomes by primary site and treatment. Results showed that significant prognostic factors varied by histologic diagnosis. For example, for nonsmall cell lung cancer and small cell lung cancer, the significant prognostic factors were KPS, age, presence of extracranial metastases, and number of brain metastases. For melanoma and renal cell cancer, the significant prognostic factors were KPS and the number of metastases. For breast and gastrointestinal (GI) cancer, the only significant prognostic factor was KPS. These data should be considered in the design of future randomized trials and in clinical decision making.

TREATMENT GUIDELINES

The modalities used to treat brain metastases include surgery, radiation, and systemic therapy, used alone or in combination.[19] The choice of which of these modalities to use is influenced by patient preference, provider preference, cost, availability, and continuing research.[20] Clinical practice parameter guidelines for the treatment of patients with metastatic brain tumors have been published with the aim of limiting variation in care without affecting clinical judgment.[21] For example, in 2010, the American Association of Neurologic Surgeons (AANS), the Congress of Neurologic Surgeons (CNS), and the Joint Tumor Section (AANS/CNS) produced multidisciplinary, evidence-linked clinical practice guidelines for the treatment of patients with metastatic brain tumors.[22] Additionally, guidelines on metastatic brain tumors have been produced by the American College of Radiology (ACR) Appropriateness Criteria and the National Cancer Institute (NCI), National Comprehensive Cancer Network (NCCN) Clinical Practice Guidelines. With general regard to all of these guidelines, patients considered to have a poor prognosis are likely to receive symptom management alone or WBRT. In contrast, patients considered to have a good prognosis are more likely to receive multimodality therapy, typically a combination of therapies aimed at local brain control, distant brain control, and systemic control.

WBRT

WBRT was the mainstay of metastatic brain tumor therapy for decades through the mid-1990s.[23] The goals of WBRT include treatment of the known metastases and prevention of future ones. The most common regimen used in North America uses parallel-opposed external beams to deliver a dose of 30 Gy, divided in a 10-dose fraction for 2 weeks.[24] Evidence suggests that altered dose/fractionation schedules of WBRT do not result in significant differences in median survival, local control, or neurocognitive outcomes when compared with standard WBRT dose/fractionation. (ie, 30 Gy in 10 fractions).[23,25]

Acute complications of WBRT include cerebral edema, nausea/vomiting, alopecia, skin reactions, and mucositis. Later complications include radiation necrosis, dementia, endocrinopathies, and diminished neurocognitive function. WBRT is often used alone in RPA class 3 patients whose alternative is best supportive care. In this setting, both overall response rate and neurologic improvement range from 50% to 60%, and survival improves from between 1 and 2 to 4 months.[26] WBRT is often used in conjunction with local treatment (surgery or stereotactic radiosurgery [SRS]) in RPA class 1/2 patients whose alternative is local treatment alone or local treatment combined with systemic treatment.[20]

SURGICAL RESECTION

The objectives of surgery include establishment of a diagnosis, local control, and rapid relief of symptoms caused by mass effect, hemorrhage, or hydrocephalus.[27] Surgery often is used in patients with RPA class 1/2, a single metastasis, and a minimal or controlled systemic tumor. Prospective surgical studies report an excellent ability to establish a diagnosis and partially improve symptoms, yet little influence on distant brain control and survival.[27] Surgical resection followed by WBRT represents a superior treatment regimen, in terms of improving tumor control at the original site of the metastasis and in the total brain, when compared with surgical resection alone. Additionally, evidence suggests that SRS alone may provide equivalent functional and survival outcomes compared with resection plus WBRT for patients with single-brain metastases, so long as ready detection of distant site failure and salvage radiotherapy are feasible.

SRS

The common objective of SRS, a convenient single outpatient procedure, is to treat single or multiple metastases and nonsurgical candidates. Tumors amenable to SRS normally measure less than 3 cm in maximum diameter and produce minimal mass effect.[28] SRS uses head immobilization, computer planning, and convergent beams to deliver a single dose of radiation with high intensity at the target and rapid dose fall-off at the margins. SRS usually is reserved for patients with a known diagnosis. According to AANS/CNS guidelines, single-dose SRS along with WBRT leads to significantly longer patient survival compared with WBRT alone for patients with single metastatic brain tumors who have a KPS greater than or equal to 70. Also, single-dose SRS along with WBRT is superior in terms of local tumor control and maintaining functional status when compared with WBRT alone for patients with one to four metastatic brain tumors who have a KPS greater than or equal to 70.[23] Retrospective and prospective studies report local control rates of 60% to 75% at 2 years, distant brain control rates of about 46% at 2 years, survival of about 10 months, decrease in the need of steroids, and trend toward survival in RPA class 1/2 patients.[29] Across retrospective studies, factors predicting distant brain control and improved outcome after SRS alone include female gender, youth, higher KPS, fewer

than three lesions, smaller total metastasis volume, surgery before SRS, nonmelanoma histology, and minimal or controlled systemic disease.[30] Otherwise and similar to surgery, there is limited impact on distant brain control and overall survival.

CHEMOTHERAPY

The primary therapeutic modality for disseminated systemic cancer remains chemotherapy.[9] Chemotherapy is used to improve local control, distant brain control, and systemic control. Chemotherapy can be used at initial diagnosis of metastatic disease or at progression.[28] It also may be used alone or in combination with radiation and can be selected either for its capacity to penetrate the blood–brain barrier (BBB) or its efficacy in specific cancer types.[31] General toxicities associated with cytotoxic chemotherapy include myelosuppression, immunosuppression, GI dysfunction, fatigue, and drug-specific toxicities.

The utility of chemotherapy in the treatment of brain metastases is limited by the BBB and by the tumor. The BBB limits the passage of large, hydrophilic molecules. Many chemotherapeutic agents are thus relatively excluded from the brain, and ones that do cross the BBB may do so in inadequate concentrations. Supporting this difficulty of crossing the BBB is the observation that intracranial radiographic response rates to chemotherapy are typically lower than extracranial radiographic response rates. An alternative hypothesis for this finding is that patients are exposed to cytotoxic therapies for their systemic disease, and it is therefore chemoresistant tumors that spread to the brain. However, data in newly diagnosed, previously untreated patients with small cell lung cancer (SCLC) suggest that intracranial response rates remain significantly lower than extracranial response rates, thereby suggesting that chemoresistant tumors do not explain this issue in full.[32] Furthermore, agents that affect peritumoral edema or CNS vasculature, including steroids and vascular endothelial growth factor (VEGF) inhibitors, may partially and temporarily affect the BBB and affect the ability to appropriately interpret imaging. Tumor-related factors also limit the usefulness of chemotherapy, including their relative size, number, chemosensitivity, and heterogeneity within the tumor itself.

Taking these factors into account, the influence or direct role of chemotherapy in patients with brain metastases is difficult to determine. Defining chemotherapy's role is further made challenging by the limited number of studies conducted, most of which are in patients with NSCLC and thus cannot be extrapolated to other histologies with confidence. Also, many studies include patients with various tumor types, uncontrolled systemic disease, undefined numbers of prior recurrences or treatments, and subjectivity in the assessment of progression and imaging response.[1] Confounding the conclusions further is the fact that some of these patients were pretreated with chemotherapy, whereas others were chemotherapy-naïve. End points also vary between studies, with some unable to reach a statistically significant conclusion with regard to a primary end point, such as survival, while reporting significant differences in other secondary end points, such as tumor radiographic response.

Many studies have looked at administering chemotherapy concurrently, before or after radiotherapy or sometimes alone. The optimal role and timing of combination therapy remain undefined. What follows is a succinct review of chemotherapy studies done to date in the context of the four most common designs in which chemotherapy has been studied in patients with brain metastases:

1. WBRT plus chemotherapy versus WBRT alone
2. Chemotherapy plus WBRT versus chemotherapy
3. Chemotherapy with concomitant WBRT versus chemotherapy with delayed WBRT
4. Chemotherapy first followed by WBRT versus WBRT first followed by chemotherapy.

Again, the role of chemotherapy in patients with brain metastases remains ill-defined, and the following review will allow the reader to better understand why.

WBRT Plus Chemotherapy versus WBRT Alone

Several chemotherapy agents have been evaluated for combination with radiation, including nitrosoureas, platinums, 5-fluorouracil agents, etoposide, topotecan, and temozolomide. To date, temozolomide has been one of the most extensively studied because of its penetration through the BBB. For example, in 2002, Antonadou and colleagues[33] conducted a phase 2 trial in which patients with brain metastases were randomized to WBRT alone or WBRT plus temozolomide. Adult patients aged 18 or older, with brain metastases from cancer of the lung, breast, or unknown primary, were included. Patients either received 40 Gy of WBRT in 20 fractions of 2 Gy each or received the same dose of WBRT with 75 mg/m^2/d of temozolomide orally during WBRT and continued temozolomide therapy (200 mg/m^2/d for 5 days every 28 days) for an additional 6 cycles after WBRT. The two

groups were similar with respect to gender, age, KPS, neurologic functional level, and tumor type. The study end points were radiographic response, neurologic symptom evaluation, and survival. The median survival was 7 months in the WBRT alone group and 8.6 months for the combination group, which was not statistically significant. The overall response rate was 67% versus 96% for WBRT alone versus combination, which was statistically significant. There was neurologic improvement in the group receiving temozolomide, with fewer patients needing corticosteroids in this same group.

In 2003, Verger and colleagues[34] conducted a phase 2 trial in patients with brain metastases randomized to WBRT alone or WBRT plus temozolomide. Adult patients aged 18 or older with a KPS greater than or equal to 50 were included. Exclusion factors included previous chemotherapy within the previous 3 weeks, prior cranial radiotherapy, and leptomeningeal involvement. Patients either received 30 Gy WBRT in 10 fractions of 3 Gy or received the same dose of WBRT with 75 mg/m^2/d of temozolomide orally during WBRT and continued temozolomide therapy (150–200 mg/m^2/d for 5 days every 28 days) for an additional 2 cycles after WBRT. The primary outcome was an analysis of neurologic toxicity, but radiologic response and progression-free survival were analyzed. The trial was stopped prematurely because of low patient accrual. The median survival was 3.1 months versus 4.5 months for WBRT alone versus combination and was not statistically significant. The overall response at day 30 was 32% for both groups. There was a statistically significant difference in cause of death between the two groups, with neurologic death occurring in 69% of patients in the WBRT alone cohort compared with 41% of patients in the WBRT plus temozolomide group.

In 2008, a single-institution phase 2 clinical trial examined the efficacy of a dose-intensified, protracted course of temozolomide (TMZ) after WBRT.[35] Patients were eligible if they had at least one bidimensionally measurable brain metastasis from breast cancer or NSCLC. Twenty-seven patients were treated with 30 Gy of WBRT with concomitant TMZ (75 mg/m^2/d) for 10 days, and subsequent TMZ at a dose of 75 mg/m^2/d for 21 days every 4 weeks, for up to 12 cycles. Two complete responses (7.4%) and 11 partial responses (40.7%) were achieved. The overall median survival was 8.8 months, and the median progression-free survival was 6 months. Authors concluded that the concomitant use of WBRT and protracted low-dose TMZ appeared to be an active, well-tolerated regimen.

In this context, other chemotherapies have been studied also. In 2004, Guerrieri and colleagues[36] published a multi-institutional, randomized controlled trial of palliative radiation with concomitant carboplatin for patients with brain metastases from NSCLC. Overall survival was the primary end point. Prior chemotherapy and prior brain radiotherapy were exclusion criteria. Forty-two patients were randomized to two groups: WBRT or WBRT plus carboplatin. The radiotherapy dose was 20 Gy in 5 fractions in both arms, and the carboplatin dose was 70 mg/m^2/d intravenously for 5 days. Unfortunately, the trial was terminated early because of low patient accrual, thus limiting the ability to draw statistically significant conclusions. The median survival was comparable, 4.4 months for WBRT versus 3.7 months for WBRT plus carboplatin, which was not statistically significant. In 2005, Kim and colleagues[37] published a retrospective cohort study that included NSCLC patients with brain metastases who received WBRT for intracranial lesions or WBRT plus platinum-based chemotherapy. The exclusion criteria were patients who did not receive WBRT. The WBRT dose was 30 to 40 Gy, and several platinum doublets were employed. There was a marked difference in median survival, WBRT alone: 19.0 weeks versus WBRT plus chemotherapy: 58.1 weeks (P<.001).

WBRT Plus Chemotherapy versus Chemotherapy

Under this design category, in 2000 a phase 3 randomized study compared teniposide versus teniposide with WBRT in patients with brain metastases from SCLC.[38] The primary end point was survival. Teniposide was administered intravenously at 120 mg/m^2 on days 1, 3, and 5 every 3 weeks up to a maximum of 12 courses or until disease progression either inside or outside the brain. WBRT, dosed at 30 Gy in 10 fractions over 2 weeks, had to be started within 3 weeks of the start of treatment with teniposide. Although the response rate in the combined modality group was significantly higher (57%) than in the teniposide alone group (22%), this did not result in a prolongation of survival, thought to be due to progression of disease outside the brain.

In 2003, Mornex and colleagues[20] performed a prospective randomized phase 3 trial of fotemustine plus WBRT versus fotemustine alone in patients with cerebral metastases from malignant melanoma. The main end points were objective response and time to cerebral progression. Patients were required to have received no chemotherapy in the prior 4 weeks, no previous nitrosourea-based chemotherapy, and no previous cerebral radiotherapy. The dose of WBRT was 37.5 Gy in 15 fractions over 3 weeks. Fotemustine was given intravenously at 100 mg/m^2 on days 1, 8, and 15, followed by a 5-week rest period and then every 3 weeks in nonprogressing patients. Although the fotemustine-alone patients had somewhat worse prognostic factors, there was no difference in cerebral response or control or in overall survival. There was a statistically significant difference in time to cerebral progression favoring the WBRT plus fotemustine group, with that group having a median time to objective cerebral progression of 56 days compared with 49 days in the chemotherapy-alone group.

Chemotherapy with Concomitant WBRT versus Chemotherapy with Delayed WBRT

Robinet and colleagues[39] conducted a randomized trial in 1998 evaluating the use of systemic chemotherapy for the treatment of inoperable brain metastases from NSCLC with early WBRT versus WBRT delayed until progression. They treated 85 patients with cisplatin and vinorelbine concurrently with WBRT and 86 with the same chemotherapy, but with WBRT delayed for at least two cycles. Patients had histologically verified NSCLC and at least one brain metastasis greater than 10 mm in diameter. Patients were treated with cisplatin 100 mg/m^2 on day 1, vinorelbine 30 mg/m^2 on days 1, 8, 15, and 22, with cycles repeated every 4 weeks. In one group, chemotherapy was started concurrent with WBRT, administered as 30 Gy in 10 fractions of 3 Gy given over 2 weeks. In the other group, radiation was deferred. The primary outcome reported was survival, for which there was no significant difference between the groups. The secondary endpoint of radiographic response was also similar, at 20% in both groups. Neurologic cause of death was reported as 88% in the group with delayed WBRT as opposed to 81% in the group treated with concurrent WBRT and chemotherapy. This study remains the only study to have attempted to answer the question of concurrent versus delayed WBRT with chemotherapy.

Chemotherapy Followed by WBRT versus WBRT Followed by Chemotherapy

Lee and colleagues[40] performed a randomized trial in 2008 examining the use of chemotherapy followed by WBRT versus WBRT followed by chemotherapy for the treatment of advanced NSCLC with brain metastases. They treated 25 patients with gemcitabine and vinorelbine before

WBRT; 23 patients were treated with WBRT followed by the same chemotherapy. Eligible patients were 18 to 75 years of age and had measurable disease in both intracranial and extracranial sites. The dose of gemcitabine was 900 mg/m² on day 1, and vinorelbine was 25 mg/m² on days 1 and 8, every 3 weeks, with a maximum of 6 cycles or disease progression. WBRT was administered as 30 Gy in 10 fractions of 3 Gy given over 10 days. In the WBRT-first arm, chemotherapy was initiated after at least a 2-week rest period. In the primary chemotherapy arm, all patients received WBRT after systemic disease progression or six cycles. There was no difference in overall response rates between the two arms (39% vs 28%, WBRT-first vs chemotherapy first). With a median follow-up of 40 months, there was no difference in progression-free survival or overall survival.

Chemotherapy Synopsis

There are other small and heterogeneous studies evaluating chemotherapy in patients with brain metastases other than what has been discussed.[1,41–44] However, even including these other studies, there remains insufficient evidence to make definitive chemotherapy recommendations in patients with newly diagnosed or recurrent/progressive brain metastases. Chemotherapy should be individualized based on a patient's functional status, extent of disease, volume and number of metastases, recurrence or progression at original versus nonoriginal site, previous treatment, and type of primary cancer. Enrollment in clinical trials is encouraged. Chemotherapy has been demonstrated to improve response rates when used as an adjunct to radiation therapy; however, these improvements in response rates have not been correlated with an improvement in median survival.[45]

NOVEL AGENTS

Several novel chemotherapy agents have been tested in patients with brain metastases. For example, gefitinib, which inhibits numerous tyrosine kinases, including the epidermal growth factor receptor (EGFR), has been used in a few NSCLC brain metastases trials; it appears to result in a partial response or stable disease in 80% to 90% of patients with brain metastases caused by NSCLC. These studies are mostly case reports and one small single arm prospective study of gefitinib for patients with brain metastases from NSCLC.[46–50] Gefitinib has not been used in patients as first-line treatment for symptomatic

brain metastases, and there is no evidence that it should be used instead of WBRT.

Agents targeting the angiogenesis pathway also have been examined in patients with brain metastases. Bevacizumab is a monoclonal antibody against vascular epidermal growth factor (VEGF). Elevated VEGFR has been linked with development of brain metastases in murine models of NSCLC.[51] To date, there are no prospective studies of antiangiogenesis agents for brain metastases in people in part because of concern regarding the possibility of treatment-related intracranial hemorrhage. Recent evidence, however, supports that bevacizumab is safe in patients with brain metastases. Besse and colleagues[52] evaluated patients who had been randomly assigned to one of 13 systemic tumor trials involving bevacizumab; these patients were subsequently diagnosed with metastases to the brain. The study showed that the patients with CNS metastases are at similar risk of developing cerebral hemorrhage, independent of bevacizumab therapy. Consequently, the authors concluded that such patients with CNS metastases from advanced/metastatic breast cancer, nonsmall cell lung carcinoma, and renal and colorectal cancer should not be excluded from bevacizumab therapy or clinical trials. Socinski and colleagues[53] recently reported on nonsmall cell lung cancer patients with previously diagnosed and treated brain metastases who subsequently safely received bevacizumab-containing treatments. Further studies are in the planning stages.

Agents related to EGFR or VEGF are not the only candidates for the targeted therapies of brain metastases. Larger prospective studies, perhaps combined with more standard therapies, will be necessary to determine if such targeted agents contribute to improved survival. Novel biologic agents like lapatinib are being investigated in the treatment of brain metastases from breast cancer with promising results.[54] Additionally, a subgroup analysis of a large prospective randomized controlled trial examining the role of radiation sensitizers suggested a prolongation of time to neurologic progression with the early use of motexafin-gadolinium (MGd).[55,56]

SYMPTOM MANAGEMENT: CORTICOSTEROIDS AND ANTICONVULSANTS

Symptom management includes the prevention and treatment of physical, cognitive, and emotional symptoms that result from both the tumor and treatment.[57] Pain, infection, deep vein thrombosis, and neurologic, cognitive, and emotional dysfunction need to be followed and treated as appropriate in relation to the etiology. For example, deficits associated with cerebral edema and consequent mass effect generally are treated with dexamethasone, which reduces cerebral edema.[58] A common cause of cerebral edema is radiation-related necrosis, which can be a complication of any form of radiation; it may be treated with surgical resection with consequent decompression, steroids, hyperbaric oxygen, or even VEGF inhibitors. Dexamethasone is the corticosteroid of choice because of its limited mineralocorticoid effects.[59] It is generally tapered slowly over several weeks to avoid rebound symptoms and adrenal insufficiency. While a great number of patients receive steroids, the medical literature contains relatively few reports addressing this issue. Dosing is generally accepted to be sufficient at twice daily, although more frequent dosing is used when there is concern for increased intracranial pressure and herniation.[60] It is important to note that based on a study by Hempen and colleagues,[61] asymptomatic patients do not need to be treated with prophylactic steroids. In this study, Hempen and colleagues retrospectively reviewed 138 consecutive patients to evaluate the impact of dosage and duration of dexamethasone administration during radiation therapy for patients with both primary and metastatic brain tumors. The dosage of dexamethasone was gradually reduced from an initial median dose of 7 to 12 mg/d to a median of 1 to 6 mg/d with an average duration of 7 weeks for the metastatic group. The authors reported that as dexamethasone was continued past a few weeks, less symptom relief was observed with increasing toxicity. Adverse effects attributed to steroid use included hyperglycemia, peripheral edema, psychiatric disorders, candidiasis, Cushing syndrome, and myopathy. The authors conclude the toxicity of dexamethasone was noted to increase over time, and therefore a patient-specific dosing pattern and taper was recommended. Gaspar and colleagues[60] published an American College of Radiology (ACR) Committee on Appropriateness Criteria consensus report following an expert panel review on the preirradiation evaluation and management of brain metastases. This consensus review indicates that the patient who shows evidence of elevated intracranial pressure, but who does not require immediate surgical attention for either hydrocephalus or impending herniation, should receive 4 to 6 mg/d of dexamethasone in divided doses and that the routine use of corticosteroids in patients without neurologic symptoms is not necessary. Looking forward in terms of additional studies in patients with brain metastases there should be a standard approach to steroid dose

and better reporting of dosages so that one may better assess symptom response and its durability. Studies also should report side effects of steroid use and the ability to taper off steroids after treatment intervention.

Anticonvulsants should be used for patients with brain metastases who have seizures. The prophylactic use of anticonvulsants in the perioperative or other settings remains controversial. Compared with the frequent use of anticonvulsants for prophylactic and active treatment of seizures associated with metastatic brain disease, the medical literature contains few reports addressing their use and efficacy. It appears as though there is no benefit from the routine prophylactic use of anticonvulsants. For example, Forsyth and colleagues[62] conducted a clinical trial to determine if prophylactic anticonvulsants in brain tumor patients (without prior seizures) reduced seizure frequency in 100 patients with newly diagnosed brain tumors. Patients were stratified for primary or metastatic histology. Of patients with brain metastasis, 26 were treated with anticonvulsants; 34 patients received no anticonvulsants. The primary outcome reported was seizure occurrence at 3 months after randomization. The trial was halted early because the seizure rate in the no anticonvulsant arm was only 10%, which put the anticipated seizure rate of 20% outside the 95% confidence interval. The only outcome reported specifically for the subgroup of patients with brain metastases was seizure incidence, and there was no significant difference between those who received anticonvulsant prophylaxis and those who did not. As such, most current guidelines have recommended against the prophylactic use of anticonvulsants.[63] Once a seizure has occurred, anticonvulsants should be used. Unresolved questions include the prognosis for patients with a single perioperative seizure versus multiple symptomatic seizures, with regards to long-term control, adverse effects of therapy, and safety.

SUMMARY

Management of brain metastases requires synchronized control of the existing metastases (local control), prevention of future metastases elsewhere in the brain (distant control), and control of the systemic cancer (systemic control). Modalities available to achieve this include WBRT, surgery, SRS, and medical therapies, such as chemotherapies and novel agents. At present, there is a lack of a clear survival benefit with the addition of chemotherapy to WBRT. Similarly, the timing question of when chemotherapy should be administered remains unanswered. At present, the selection of the combination of these treatment measures remains highly individualized and influenced by factors involving the tumor, patient, provider, and treatment guidelines. Future treatment advances will require a multidisciplinary approach integrating surgical, radiation, and chemotherapeutic options to improve neurologic function and quality of life, rather than just focusing on survival endpoints.

For now, patients and physicians alike must weigh the risks and potential symptoms of both the recurrence of the tumor and the complications of treatment. Chief among these concerns for future studies is diminished neurocognitive function associated with WBRT. Until recently, most studies did not routinely evaluate neurocognitive domains of attention, information processing, memory, verbal fluency, executive function, or fine motor skills. However, recent studies have begun to comprehensively examine the impact of tumor burden, tumor recurrence, and treatment on neurocognitive function.

REFERENCES

1. Walbert T, Gilbert MR. The role of chemotherapy in the treatment of patients with brain metastases from solid tumors. Int J Clin Oncol 2009;14(4): 299–306.
2. Gavrilovic IT, Posner JB. Brain metastases: epidemiology and pathophysiology. J Neurooncol 2005; 75(1):5–14.
3. Chamberlain MC. Brain metastases: a medical neuro-oncology perspective. Expert Rev Neurother 2010;10(4):563–73.
4. Norden AD, Wen PY, Kesari S. Brain metastases. Curr Opin Neurol 2005;18(6):654–61.
5. Ammirati M, et al. The role of retreatment in the management of recurrent/progressive brain metastases: a systematic review and evidence-based clinical practice guideline. J Neurooncol 2010;96(1): 85–96.
6. Robinson PD, et al. Methodology used to develop the AANS/CNS management of brain metastases evidence-based clinical practice parameter guidelines. J Neurooncol 2010;96(1):11–6.
7. Sperduto PW, et al. Diagnosis-specific prognostic factors, indexes, and treatment outcomes for patients with newly diagnosed brain metastases: a multi-institutional analysis of 4259 patients. Int J Radiat Oncol Biol Phys 2010;77(3):655–61.
8. Soffietti R, Ruda R, Trevisan E. Brain metastases: current management and new developments. Curr Opin Oncol 2008;20(6):676–84.
9. Yamanaka R. Medical management of brain metastases from lung cancer. Oncol Rep 2009;22(6): 1269–76.
10. Soffietti R, Ruda R, Mutani R. Management of brain metastases. J Neurol 2002;249(10):1357–69.
11. Lee SS, et al. Brain metastases in breast cancer: prognostic factors and management. Breast Cancer Res Treat 2008;111(3):523–30.
12. Lagerwaard FJ, et al. Identification of prognostic factors in patients with brain metastases: a review of 1292 patients. Int J Radiat Oncol Biol Phys 1999;43(4):795–803.
13. Meier S, et al. Survival and prognostic factors in patients with brain metastases from malignant melanoma. Onkologie 2004;27(2):145–9.
14. Golden DW, et al. Prognostic factors and grading systems for overall survival in patients treated with radiosurgery for brain metastases: variation by primary site. J Neurosurg 2008;109:77–86.
15. Chidel MA, et al. Application of recursive partitioning analysis and evaluation of the use of whole brain radiation among patients treated with stereotactic radiosurgery for newly diagnosed brain metastases. Int J Radiat Oncol Biol Phys 2000;47(4):993–9.
16. Gaspar L, et al. Recursive partitioning analysis (RPA) of prognostic factors in three Radiation Therapy Oncology Group (RTOG) brain metastases trials. Int J Radiat Oncol Biol Phys 1997;37(4): 745–51.
17. Thomas SS, Dunbar EM. Modern multidisciplinary management of brain metastases. Curr Oncol Rep 2010;12(1):34–40.
18. Sperduto PW, et al. A new prognostic index and comparison to three other indices for patients with brain metastases: an analysis of 1960 patients in the RTOG database. Int J Radiat Oncol Biol Phys 2008;70(2):510–4.
19. Ewend MG, et al. Guidelines for the initial management of metastatic brain tumors: role of surgery, radiosurgery, and radiation therapy. J Natl Compr Canc Netw 2008;6(5):505–13 [quiz: 514].
20. Mornex F, et al. A prospective randomized multi-centre phase III trial of fotemustine plus whole brain irradiation versus fotemustine alone in cerebral metastases of malignant melanoma. Melanoma Res 2003;13(1):97–103.
21. Soffietti R, et al. EFNS Guidelines on diagnosis and treatment of brain metastases: report of an EFNS Task Force. Eur J Neurol 2006;13(7):674–81.
22. Linskey ME, Kalkanis SN. Evidence-linked, clinical practice guidelines—getting serious; getting professional. J Neurooncol 2010;96(1):1–5.
23. Gaspar LE, et al. The role of whole brain radiation therapy in the management of newly diagnosed brain metastases: a systematic review and evidence-based clinical practice guideline. J Neurooncol 2010;96(1):17–32.
24. Mintz A, et al. Management of single brain metastasis: a practice guideline. Curr Oncol 2007;14(4): 131–43.

25. Tsao MN, et al. Whole-brain radiotherapy for the treatment of multiple brain metastases. Cochrane Database Syst Rev 2006;3:CD003869.

26. Nieder C, Berberich W, Schnabel K. Tumor-related prognostic factors for remission of brain metastases after radiotherapy. Int J Radiat Oncol Biol Phys 1997;39(1):25–30.

27. Kalkanis SN, et al. The role of surgical resection in the management of newly diagnosed brain metastases: a systematic review and evidence-based clinical practice guideline. J Neurooncol 2010;96(1): 33–43.

28. Linskey ME, et al. The role of stereotactic radiosurgery in the management of patients with newly diagnosed brain metastases: a systematic review and evidence-based clinical practice guideline. J Neurooncol 2010;96(1):45–68.

29. Andrews DW, et al. Whole-brain radiation therapy with or without stereotactic radiosurgery boost for patients with one to three brain metastases: phase III results of the RTOG 9508 randomised trial. Lancet 2004;363(9422):1665–72.

30. Sawrie SM, et al. Predictors of distant brain recurrence for patients with newly diagnosed brain metastases treated with stereotactic radiosurgery alone. Int J Radiat Oncol Biol Phys 2008;70(1):181–6.

31. Gerstner ER, Fine RL. Increased permeability of the blood-brain barrier to chemotherapy in metastatic brain tumors: establishing a treatment paradigm. J Clin Oncol 2007;25(16):2306–12.

32. Seute T, et al. Response of asymptomatic brain metastases from small-cell lung cancer to systemic first-line chemotherapy. J Clin Oncol 2006;24(13): 2079–83.

33. Antonadou D, et al. Phase II randomized trial of temozolomide and concurrent radiotherapy in patients with brain metastases. J Clin Oncol 2002;20(17): 3644–50.

34. Verger E, et al. Temozolomide and concomitant whole brain radiotherapy in patients with brain metastases: a phase II randomized trial. Int J Radiat Oncol Biol Phys 2005;61(1):185–91.

35. Addeo R, et al. Phase 2 trial of temozolomide using protracted low-dose and whole-brain radiotherapy for nonsmall cell lung cancer and breast cancer patients with brain metastases. Cancer 2008;113(9): 2524–31.

36. Guerrieri M, et al. A randomised phase III study of palliative radiation with concomitant carboplatin for brain metastases from non-small cell carcinoma of the lung. Lung Cancer 2004;46(1):107–11.

37. Kim DY, et al. Efficacy of platinum-based chemotherapy after cranial radiation in patients with brain metastasis from nonsmall cell lung cancer. Oncol Rep 2005;14(1):207–11.

38. Postmus PE, et al. Treatment of brain metastases of small-cell lung cancer: comparing teniposide and teniposide with whole-brain radiotherapy—a phase III study of the European Organization for the Research and Treatment of Cancer Lung Cancer Cooperative Group. J Clin Oncol 2000;18(19): 3400–8.

39. Robinet G, et al. Results of a phase III study of early versus delayed whole brain radiotherapy with concurrent cisplatin and vinorelbine combination in inoperable brain metastasis of nonsmall cell lung cancer: Groupe Francais de Pneumo-Cancerologie (GFPC) Protocol 95-1. Ann Oncol 2001;12(1):59–67.

40. Lee DH, et al. Primary chemotherapy for newly diagnosed nonsmall cell lung cancer patients with synchronous brain metastases compared with whole-brain radiotherapy administered first: result of a randomized pilot study. Cancer 2008;113(1): 143–9.

41. McWilliams RR, et al. Melanoma-induced brain metastases. Expert Rev Anticancer Ther 2008;8(5): 743–55.

42. Schild SE, et al. Brain metastases from melanoma: is there a role for concurrent temozolomide in addition to whole brain radiation therapy? Am J Clin Oncol 2009.

43. Mehta MP, et al. The role of chemotherapy in the management of newly diagnosed brain metastases: a systematic review and evidence-based clinical practice guideline. J Neurooncol 2010;96(1):71–83.

44. Olson JJ, et al. The role of emerging and investigational therapies for metastatic brain tumors: a systematic review and evidence-based clinical practice guideline of selected topics. J Neurooncol 2010;96(1):115–42.

45. Peacock KH, Lesser GJ. Current therapeutic approaches in patients with brain metastases. Curr Treat Options Oncol 2006;7(6):479–89.

46. Shimato S, et al. EGFR mutations in patients with brain metastases from lung cancer: association with the efficacy of gefitinib. Neuro Oncol 2006; 8(2):137–44.

47. Namba Y, et al. Gefitinib in patients with brain metastases from nonsmall cell lung cancer: review of 15 clinical cases. Clin Lung Cancer 2004;6(2): 123–8.

48. Hotta K, et al. Effect of gefitinib (Iressa, ZD1839) on brain metastases in patients with advanced nonsmall cell lung cancer. Lung Cancer 2004;46(2): 255–61.

49. Ceresoli GL, et al. Gefitinib in patients with brain metastases from nonsmall cell lung cancer: a prospective trial. Ann Oncol 2004;15(7):1042–7.

50. Chiu CH, et al. Gefitinib is active in patients with brain metastases from nonsmall cell lung cancer and response is related to skin toxicity. Lung Cancer 2005;47(1):129–38.

51. Yano S, et al. Expression of vascular endothelial growth factor is necessary but not sufficient for

production and growth of brain metastasis. Cancer Res 2000;60(17):4959–67.

52. Besse B, et al. Bevacizumab safety in patients with central nervous system metastases. Clin Cancer Res 2010;16(1):269–78.

53. Socinski MA, et al. Safety of bevacizumab in patients with nonsmall cell lung cancer and brain metastases. J Clin Oncol 2009;27(31):5255–61.

54. Arslan C, Dizdar O, Altundag K. Systemic treatment in breast-cancer patients with brain metastasis. Expert Opin Pharmacother 2010;11(7):1089–100.

55. Ryken TC, et al. The role of steroids in the management of brain metastases: a systematic review and evidence-based clinical practice guideline. J Neurooncol 2010;96(1):103–14.

56. Ricciardi S, de Marinis F. Multimodality management of nonsmall cell lung cancer patients with brain metastases. Curr Opin Oncol 2010;22(2):86–93.

57. Kaal EC, Taphoorn MJ, Vecht CJ. Symptomatic management and imaging of brain metastases. J Neurooncol 2005;75(1):15–20.

58. Koehler PJ. Use of corticosteroids in neuro-oncology. Anticancer Drugs 1995;6(1):19–33.

59. Mikkelsen T, et al. The role of prophylactic anticonvulsants in the management of brain metastases: a systematic review and evidence-based clinical practice guideline. J Neurooncol 2010;96(1):97–102.

60. Gaspar LE, et al. Preisrradiation evaluation and management of brain metastases. American College of Radiology. ACR appropriateness criteria. Radiology 2000;215:1105–10.

61. Hempen C, Weiss E, Hess CF. Dexamethasone treatment in patients with brain metastases and primary brain tumors: do the benefits outweigh the side effects? Support Care Cancer 2002;10(4):322–8.

62. Forsyth PA, et al. Prophylactic anticonvulsants in patients with brain tumour. Can J Neurol Sci 2003;30(2):106–12.

63. Glantz MJ, et al. Practice parameter: anticonvulsant prophylaxis in patients with newly diagnosed brain tumors. Report of the Quality Standards Subcommittee of the American Academy of Neurology. Neurology 2000;54(10):1886–93.

Radiotherapy for Brain Metastases

Robert B. Den, MD[a], David W. Andrews, MD[b],*

KEYWORDS

• Brain metastases • Treatment approaches • SRS • WBRT

The optimal treatment of brain metastases remains controversial. There are several patient- and treatment-related factors that must be considered to determine the optimal management for a given patient. At present, there is randomized control evidence supporting multiple treatment strategies incorporating radiotherapy.

INCIDENCE

Brain metastases affect 20% to 40% of patients with cancer[1] and are the most common intracranial tumor in adults. The incidence of metastases is thought to be increasing because of better detection and treatment of systemic malignancy. When considering various treatment approaches for brain metastases it is crucial to distinguish between single metastasis, only one lesion in the brain, regardless of extracranial status, and solitary metastasis, central nervous system (CNS) metastasis as the only site of disease, because this has disparate prognostic significance.

PROGNOSIS

In 1997, the Radiation Therapy Oncology Group (RTOG) analyzed their database of 1200 patients with brain metastases from 3 consecutive RTOG trials conducted between 1979 and 1993 to determine the patient factors that affected overall survival (OS).[2] This report defined 3 groups by recursive partitioning analysis (RPA): group 1, patients with Karnofsky performance score (KPS) of 70 or more, age less than 65 years, primary controlled metastasis, and no other extracranial metastasis; group 2, patients with KPS of 70 or more, age of 65 years or greater, primary uncontrolled metastasis, other extracranial metastases; and group 3, patients with KPS less than 70. The median OS for these 3 cohorts was 7.1 months, 4.2 months, and 2.3 months, respectively.

Since the publication of the report, there have been 2 updates to the RTOG RPA classification. Sperduto and colleagues[3] devised a new classification called the graded prognostic assessment (GPA) based on the RPA classification. The advantage of the GPA over the RPA classification is its ease of use and objectivity. The GPA classification is developed based on a point system and uses the following criteria: age, KPS, and cranial and extracranial metastases. Patient age is scored (0, 0.5, 1) stratified by age greater than 60 years, 50 to 59 years, or less than 50 years. KPS is scored (0, 0.5, 1) for age less than 70 years, 70 to 80 years, and 90 to 100 years. Cranial metastases are scored (0, 0.5, 1) for 3 brain metastases, 2 to 3 brain metastases, and 1 brain metastasis. Extracranial metastases are scored (0 or 1) if present or absent. The scores are summed, and OS correlates with higher score. Median OS is 2.6 months, 3.8 months, 6.9 months, and 11.0 months for a GPA score of 0 to 1, 1.5 to 2.5, 3, and 3.5 to 4, respectively.

In addition, the RTOG recently defined disease-specific GPA[4] based on more than 4000 patients with newly diagnosed brain metastases. This study defined various prognostic factors, which were scored to categorize patients based on OS. For patients with lung cancer (both small cell lung cancer [SCLC] and non-SCLC [NSCLC]), 4 prognostic factors were included (age, KPS, extracranial metastases, and number of brain metastases). For

[a] Department of Radiation Oncology, Thomas Jefferson University, 111 South 11th Street, Bodine Cancer Center, Philadelphia, PA 19107, USA
[b] Department of Neurosurgery, Thomas Jefferson University, 909 Walnut Street, 3rd Floor, Philadelphia, PA 19107, USA
* Corresponding author.
E-mail address: david.andrews@jefferson.edu

Neurosurg Clin N Am 22 (2011) 37–44
doi:10.1016/j.nec.2010.08.001
1042-3680/11/$ — see front matter. Published by Elsevier Inc.

patients with renal cell carcinoma or melanoma, 2 prognostic factors were used (KPS and number of brain metastases). For brain metastases from either a mammillary or gastrointestinal source, only KPS was required for prognostic significance. Based on these patient factors, median OS was determined (**Tables 1** and **2**).

NATURAL HISTORY

The natural history of symptomatic brain metastases is severe without surgical or radiotherapeutic intervention. The median OS without any treatment is 1 month[5] and with glucocorticosteroids alone reaches 2 months.[6] Thus, it is critical to determine a patient's expected survival before initiation of therapy; if it seems to be less than 30 days, intervention may not be warranted.

TREATMENT APPROACHES

There are several different treatment approaches for patients with brain metastases. Herein, the randomized evidence supporting various algorithms is presented. There is at present much controversy between the standard of care and the current National Comprehensive Cancer Network (NCCN) guidelines. The 2010 NCCN guidelines recommend either whole brain radiotherapy (WBRT) or chemotherapy for patients with 1 to 3 brain metastases, disseminated systemic disease, and poor treatment options. For patients with stable or newly diagnosed systemic disease with 1 to 3 brain metastases, options include surgery followed by WBRT or stereotactic radiosurgery (SRS), SRS plus WBRT, or SRS alone. For patients with greater than 3 metastases, WBRT alone is recommended.

WBRT Alone

WBRT as a monotherapy for brain metastases generally consists of opposed lateral beams covering the entire cranium with margin and treatment with a dose of 30 Gy in 10 fractions (fxns). This dose and fractionation scheme was tested in 2 RTOG trials,[7] RTOG 6901 and RTOG 7361. RTOG 6901 randomized 910 patients to 4 radiation schemes (30 Gy in 10 fxns, 30 Gy in 15 fxns, 40 Gy in 15 fxns, and 40 Gy in 20 fxns) with a median survival of 4.8, 4.1, 4.1, and 3.6 months, respectively, whereas RTOG 7361 analyzed 3 different radiation dose fractionation approaches (20 Gy in 5 fxns, 30 Gy in 10 fxns, and 40 Gy in 15 fxns) and found no difference in the median OS of 3.4, 3.6, and 3.6 months, respectively. Numerous other randomized controlled trials[8–20] compared various fractionation schemes, and none have been shown to be superior. However, RTOG 85–28[13] that delivered 32 Gy twice a day (1.6 Gy/fxn) plus an escalating boost for a total dose of 48 to 70.4 Gy showed increased survival for doses greater than 54 Gy, but these results were not validated in the subsequent RTOG 9104 trial.[9]

WBRT with or without Surgery

Having established the benefit of WBRT over steroids or no treatment in terms of OS, the role of surgical management was analyzed in 3 randomized controlled trials[21–23] and 1 trial originally randomized but changed to a registry trial because of poor accrual.[24] Patchell and colleagues[21] randomized 48 patients with suspected single brain metastasis to biopsy and then to WBRT versus surgery plus WBRT. Surgery was performed within 72 hours of randomization, and WBRT was administered within 14 days of surgery; for those patients

Table 1
GPA criteria for brain metastases

	Points					
	0	0.5	1	2	3	4
NSCLC/SCLC						
Age (y)	>60	59–50	<50			
KPS	<70	70–80	90–100			
No. of Cranial Metastases	>3	2–3	1			
Extracranial Metastases	Present		Absent			
Renal Cell Carcinoma/Melanoma						
KPS	<70	70–80	90–100			
No. of Cranial Metastases	>3	2–3	1			
Breast/Gastrointestinal Tract						
KPS	<70		70	80	90	100

Table 2
Median OS (in months)

GPA Score	NSCLC	SCLC	Melanoma	Renal Cell Carcinoma	Breast	Gastrointestinal Tract
0—1.0	3.0	2.8	3.4	3.3	6.1	3.1
1.5—2.5	6.5	5.3	4.7	7.3	9.4	4.4
3.0	11.3	9.6	8.8	11.3	16.9	6.9
3.5—4.0	14.8	17.0	13.2	14.8	18.7	13.5
Overall	7.0	4.9	6.7	9.6	11.9	5.4

randomized to WBRT alone, treatment began within 48 hours of randomization or biopsy. The dose and fractionation was 36 Gy in 12 fxns. The results revealed an increase in median OS (9 months vs 3 months, $P<.05$), decrease in "neurologic death" (14 months vs 6 months, $P<.05$), decrease in local recurrence (20% vs 52%, $P<.05$), time to recurrence (>14 months vs 5 months, $P<.05$), and quality of life for patients with KPS greater than 70 (9 months vs 2 months, $P<.05$) for surgery plus WBRT compared with WBRT alone. There was lower distant brain recurrence, 20% versus 13% ($P = .52$), and no difference in systemic death. Thus, this trial demonstrated that for patients with single metastasis, the addition of surgery to WBRT results in patients living longer, having fewer recurrences, and having improved quality of life in comparison to patients receiving WBRT alone. The second published study by Vecht and colleagues[22] randomized 63 patients with suspected single brain metastasis to resection plus WBRT versus WBRT alone. The WBRT dosage was 2 Gy twice a day for 40 Gy over 2 weeks. None of the patients underwent magnetic resonance imaging (MRI) staging. This study showed that the median OS improved with WBRT plus surgery compared with WBRT alone (10 months vs 6 months, $P<.05$). For patients with stable extracranial disease, the median OS improved with surgery from 7 months to 12 months. However, in patients with progressive extracranial disease, there was no difference in the median OS between the 2 groups (median OS was 5 months for both the groups). In terms of functional independence, patients with stable extracranial disease had longer independence with surgery (4 months vs 9 months), but no difference was noted in those with progressive extracranial disease (2.5 months for both the groups). This trial demonstrated an improvement in OS for all patients; however, further analysis revealed that most deaths were caused by systemic disease and surgery benefited those with stable extracranial disease. The third randomized trial by Mintz and colleagues[23] randomized 84 patients with suspected single brain metastasis and KPS

greater than 50 to WBRT (30 Gy in 10 fxns) versus WBRT plus surgery. All patients underwent computed tomographic staging. This trial failed to demonstrate an improvement in median OS for the addition of surgery to WBRT (6 months vs 6 months), and in addition, there was no difference in quality of life. However, this trial allowed patients with worse baseline KPS to be enrolled, and this population was shown to have minimal to no benefit with the addition of surgery to WBRT. Thus, the 3 randomized trials reveal a benefit to OS in patients with KPS greater than 70 with the addition of surgery to WBRT.

Surgery with or without WBRT

Having demonstrated the benefit of adding surgery to WBRT, the reverse question was explored in one randomized controlled trial. Patchell and colleagues[25] randomized 95 patients with single brain metastasis to complete resection (verified by MRI) followed by observation or postoperative WBRT (50.4 Gy over 5.5 weeks). Patients were eligible if their KPS was greater than 70, despite other sites of metastases. Randomization was stratified by the extent of extracranial disease and primary tumor type. The primary outcome was tumor recurrence anywhere in the brain. Postoperative WBRT was associated with less recurrence anywhere in the brain (18% vs 70%, $P<.05$), at the site of resection (10% vs 46%, $P<.05$), and in other areas of the brain (14% vs 37%, $P<.05$). In addition, there was decreased neurologic death (14% vs 44%, $P<.05$). There was no difference in OS or length of time for which the patient remained independent. This study was not powered to demonstrate a difference in overall time. Also, it should be noted that this study used a nonstandard WBRT dose. However, this study demonstrated a benefit in terms of neurologic death and local control to the addition of WBRT to surgery.

A second randomized controlled trial conducted by the European Organization for Research and Treatment of Cancer (EORTC) randomized patients to surgery or SRS and to observation or WBRT. This work has been presented as an abstract at the 2009 American Society of Therapeutic Radiation Oncology annual meeting. EORTC 22952-26001[26] randomized 359 patients with 1 to 3 brain metastases, with or without stable systemic disease or asymptomatic primary tumors, and KPS from 0 to 2 to surgery (160 patients) or SRS (185 patients) and to observation or WBRT (30 Gy in 10 fxns). Within the surgical arm, 96% of patients had solitary lesions, whereas in the SRS arm, 33% had multiple lesions. The median survival was 10 months (observation) versus 9.5 months (WBRT), which was not a statistically significant difference. Intracranial progression at 6 months and 24 months was 39.7% and 54.2% versus 15.2% and 31.2% for observation and WBRT, respectively. Statistically significant reduction was there in local failure (31.3% vs 16.4%) as well as distant intracranial failures (32.4% vs 17.6%) (P<.001). In addition, neurologic cause of death was 43% versus 25%. The results of this study are similar to the prior trials in that there is no improvement in OS with WBRT; however, it demonstrated improvement in local control, distant intracranial failure, and death from neurologic causes.

Role of SRS

SRS has been explored in the management of brain metastases alone or in conjunction with surgery and WBRT. There are no randomized trials of surgery with or without SRS or surgery versus SRS, and thus this topic is not discussed further. However, several trials have examined the benefit of the addition of SRS to WBRT and the converse case of addition of WBRT to SRS.

WBRT with or without SRS

WBRT with or without SRS has been studied in 2 randomized controlled trials. Andrews and colleagues[27] randomized 331 patients with 1 to 3 brain metastases with a maximum diameter of 4 cm to WBRT 37.5 Gy per 15 fxns versus WBRT plus radiosurgery (15–24 Gy, based on size) in the multicenter setting. Patients were stratified by the number of metastases and extent of extracranial disease. The primary end point was median survival. Secondary end points included tumor control at 1 year, KPS and mini-mental state examination (MMSE) at 6 months, and cause of death (neurologic vs nonneurologic). The median OS was 6.5 months versus 5.7 months for WBRT versus WBRT plus SRS, respectively (P = .14); however, for patients with single metastasis, OS was 4.9 months versus 6.5 months (P<.05). In

addition, there was a higher 3-month response rate and local control at 1 year (71% vs 82%) for the addition of SRS to WBRT. There was no difference in overall time to progression (any intracranial failure) and neurologic death. Local recurrence was 43% more likely with WBRT alone than with WBRT plus SRS. There was an improved KPS (4% vs 13%) and decreased steroid use at 6 months for WBRT plus SRS, but there was no difference in mental status. In summary, this trial demonstrated that WBRT plus SRS was beneficial for patients with single metastasis but did not improve median OS.

A second single-institution randomized controlled trial from the University of Pittsburgh led by Kondziolka and colleagues[28] randomized adults with a KPS greater than 70 with 2 to 4 solid metastatic brain tumors, each 2.5 cm in mean diameter, to WBRT versus WBRT plus SRS. The primary end point of the study was imaging-defined local control. This trial was stopped early after a significant interim benefit in local control was demonstrated for the WBRT plus SRS arm. From the 27 patients randomized, the 1-year local failure was 100% versus 8% for WBRT versus WBRT plus SRS (P<.05) and the time to failure was 6 months versus 36 months for WBRT versus WBRT plus SRS (P<.05). The median OS was 7.5 months versus 11 months (P = .22); however, because of early termination, the statistical power to assess differences in median survival was limited. However, patients in the WBRT arm who received salvage SRS had a median OS of 11 months (similar to WBRT with immediate SRS), whereas patients who received only WBRT had a median OS of 7 months (P<.05 to WBRT plus SRS). Thus, these data demonstrate a benefit to the addition of SRS to WBRT.

SRS with or without WBRT

There are 2 published, prospective, randomized trials comparing SRS alone with SRS plus WBRT,[29,30] and 1 prospective randomized trial has been presented as an abstract comparing surgery or SRS with either surgery or SRS with adjuvant WBRT.[26] The first published trial JROSG 99–1 randomized patients with 1 to 4 brain metastases, size less than 3 cm, and RPA class I to II to SRS alone (for <2 cm, 22–25 Gy; for 2–3 cm, 18–20 Gy) versus WBRT (30 Gy in 10 fxns) followed by SRS (with a dose reduction of 30%). The primary end point was OS, and the trial was terminated early (132 of expected 188 patients enrolled) because of low likelihood of showing a difference in primary end point. The trial demonstrated a median OS of 7.5 months versus 8.0

months ($P = .42$), with a discordant 1-year OS of 38% versus 28% ($P = .42$) for WBRT plus SRS versus SRS, respectively. Although neurologic death (23% vs 19% [$P = .64$] for WBRT plus SRS versus SRS alone) was not significant, there was a statistically significant difference in the 12-month actuarial local tumor control rate of 88.7% in the WBRT plus SRS group versus 72.5% in the SRS-alone group ($P = .002$), 12-month actuarial brain tumor recurrence rate of 46.8% in the WBRT plus SRS group versus 76.4% in the SRS-alone group ($P<.001$), and 12-month actuarial rate of developing new brain metastases of 41.5% in the WBRT plus SRS group versus 63.7% in the SRS-alone group ($P = .003$). Further, the addition of WBRT decreased the need for salvage brain treatment (10 patients vs 29 patients), and importantly, no statistically significant difference in neurotoxicity was reported. A more detailed review[31] of the trial's neurocognitive component as assessed by MMSE revealed that the average duration until deterioration of neurocognition was 16.5 months in the WBRT plus SRS group and 7.6 months in the SRS-alone group ($P = .05$). Thus, indicating that control of the brain tumor is the most important factor for stabilizing neurocognitive function (NCF).

The second randomized controlled study[30] was a single-institutional study that randomized patients with RPA class I to II (KPS$\geq$70) and 1 to 3 brain metastases to SRS (median dose of 19 Gy) versus SRS (median dose, 20 Gy) plus WBRT (30 Gy in 12 fxns). The primary end point of this trial was NCF that is objectively measured as a significant deterioration (5-point drop compared with baseline) in Hopkins Verbal Learning Test-Revised (HVLT-R) total recall at 4 months. This trial was halted early (58 of expected 90 patients enrolled) because of significantly worse cognitive outcome in WBRT plus SRS arm. The results of the trial revealed that OS was compromised in the WBRT plus SRS arm. The median and 1-year survival were higher for the SRS-alone group than for patients in the SRS plus WBRT group (15.2 months vs 5.7 months, 63% vs 21%; $P = .003$); however, 1-year local tumor control rate was 67% for patients in the SRS group and 100% for patients in the SRS plus WBRT group ($P = .012$), the 1-year distant brain tumor control rate was 45% for patients in the SRS group and 73% for patients in the SRS plus WBRT group ($P = .02$), and the 1-year freedom from CNS metastasis recurrence was 27% (95% confidence interval [CI], 14–51) for the SRS group and 73% (95% CI, 46–100) for the SRS plus WBRT ($P<.001$) group. Thus, in case of neurologic control, SRS plus WBRT was

superior. However, death from neurologic causes was not statistically significant (7 deaths vs 8 deaths, $P = .15$). In the SRS-alone arm, 1 patient received salvage WBRT and 7 patients underwent salvage craniotomy compared with none in the SRS plus WBRT arm. NCF had a statistically significant decline (52% vs 24%) in the SRS plus WBRT arm versus SRS-alone arm. Thus, this trial demonstrated that the addition of WBRT improved local neurologic control, distant brain disease, and freedom from CNS metastasis recurrence but failed to show an improvement in death from neurologic cause, and in fact, this trial demonstrated worse NCF and OS. This is the first trial to show a decline in OS for the addition of WBRT.

However, there are several criticisms to this trial that should be noted. A prior prospective study[32] revealed that for patients treated with WBRT a biphasic pattern of post-WBRT NCF is noted. With multiple time points measured, NCF of long-term survivors typically declines at about the 2- to 4-month point but subsequently rebounds. Given the complexity of NCF, a battery of tests over time is required to assess neurocognition adequately.[33] Another concern is the balance of the study groups. Several findings point to patients in the combined group having a disproportionately worse prognosis at outset. The SRS-alone group comprised a majority of women, patients with single metastasis, RPA class I patients, and an absence of patients with lung and abdominal metastases. In fact, the OS of the SRS-alone arm was 7 months longer than that of the Japanese study[29] (15.2 months vs 8.0 months). Furthermore, the combined therapy group had a greater burden in disease volume. Baseline NCF is highly correlated with the volume of indicator lesions but not with the number of metastases.[34] In addition, there was a trend for worse baseline function in the SRS plus WBRT arm versus SRS-alone arm. Also, the investigators did not account for possible bias due to medications, which could have adversely affected neurocognition.[35] There was a high rate of salvage in the SRS-alone arm. This finding suggests that treatment assignment led to bias in the subsequent aggressive approach to salvage therapy in the SRS-alone group. In the SRS-alone group, chemotherapy was administered to more patients and for a longer duration. Given the proximity of death to the primary end point (1-month difference), it is unclear if the decline in NCF was caused by irradiation or progressive decline. Several studies revealed a decline in mental function before death.[36]

There is currently 1 open trial examining the question of SRS with or without WBRT and it is being conducted by the North Central Cancer

Group and American College of Surgeons Oncology Group. This trial is randomizing patients with 1 to 3 cerebral metastases to SRS versus SRS plus WBRT. The primary end point is OS, and secondary end points include time to CNS (brain) failure, quality of life, duration of functional independence, long-term neurocognitive status, and posttreatment toxicity.

Can WBRT Be Improved with the Addition of Chemotherapy?

There have been several randomized controlled trials examining the addition of various chemotherapeutic agents to WBRT. None of the trials demonstrated a statistically significant improvement in OS. Phillips and colleagues[11] conducted the RTOG 8905 trial that randomized 72 patients with a KPS of 70 or more and no other metastases to WBRT (37.5 Gy/15 fxns) with or without bromodeoxyuridine. The median OS was 6.1 months versus 4.3 months ($P = .904$) for the WBRT versus WBRT plus bromodeoxyuridine groups. Mehta and colleagues[37] randomized 401 patients to 30-Gy WBRT versus WBRT with concurrent motexafin gadolinium. There was no difference in survival (4.9 months vs 5.2 months, $P = .48$) or time to neurologic progression (9.5 months vs 8.3 months, $P = .95$). However, there was an improvement in neurologic progression in patients with NSCLC. Guerrieri and colleagues[38] randomized 42 patients with brain metastases from NSCLC to WBRT with or without carboplatin. OS was 4.4 months versus 3.7 months ($P = .64$), but this trial was stopped early because of poor accrual. Ushio and colleagues[39] randomized patients with lung cancer to 3 arms, WBRT, WBRT plus chloroethylnitrosureas, and WBRT plus chloroethylnitrosureas plus tegafur. There was no difference in survival among the 3 arms. Neuhaus and colleagues[40] randomized 96 of a planned 320 patients with SCLC or NSCLC and with brain metastases to WBRT (40 Gy in 20 fxns) versus WBRT plus topotecan. This trial was closed early because of poor accrual, and there was no difference in local recurrence or disease-free survival. Knisely and colleagues[41] randomized patients in the multicenter arena on RTOG 0118 to WBRT (37.5 Gy in 15 fxns) with or without thalidomide. This trial, which was stopped early because of nonsuperiority, accrued 183 patients with multiple (>3), large (>4 cm), or midbrain metastases from extracranial disease. The median OS in both cohorts was 3.9 months; however, 48% of patients had to discontinue use of thalidomide due to toxicity. Thus, these collective studies failed to demonstrate a benefit to the addition of chemotherapy to WBRT.

Can WBRT Be Improved?

Improvement to traditional WBRT is currently being examined in the RTOG trial. Given the concern for neurocognitive decline after WBRT, an intensity-modulated hippocampal sparing approach is being pursued. RTOG 0933 is a phase 2 clinical trial that aims to test the hypothesis that for patients with brain metastases, avoiding the hippocampus during WBRT may delay or reduce the onset, frequency, and/or severity of NCF decline, without compromising intracranial disease control. Numerous studies have examined the incidence of brain metastasis within 5 mm of the hippocampal regions. Gondi and colleagues[42] found that of the more than 1000 brain metastases evaluated, 34 (3%) were within 5 mm of the hippocampus and none were in the hippocampus. Thus, the feasibility of improving memory decline without compromising function is possible.

Another approach to reduce neurocognitive decline being pursued in the prospective setting is the addition of memantine, an N-methyl-D-aspartate receptor antagonist that has proven to be effective in the treatment of vascular dementia, to WBRT in RTOG 0614. This trial randomizes patients to WBRT (37.5 Gy in 15 fxns) versus placebo or memantine. The planned accrual is 536 patients, and the primary outcome is to determine whether the addition of memantine to WBRT preserves NCF, specifically memory as measured by the HVLT-R for delayed recall, compared with placebo and WBRT in patients with brain metastases at 24 weeks from the beginning of drug treatment.

SUMMARY

There is a clear benefit to the addition of radiotherapy in the management of brain metastases. WBRT has been shown to be beneficial when added to surgery, and surgery has been demonstrated to be beneficial to WBRT in patients with good KPS and controlled extracranial disease. The role of WBRT followed by SRS has been demonstrated to provide benefit including improvement of OS, but SRS followed by WBRT continues to remain controversial. There are several trials that examine improving the neurotoxicity associated with WBRT. However, there is no role to the addition of chemotherapy to WBRT at present.

REFERENCES

1. Gavrilovic IT, Posner JB. Brain metastases: epidemiology and pathophysiology. J Neurooncol 2005;75: 5–14.
2. Gaspar L, Scott C, Rotman M, et al. Recursive partitioning analysis (RPA) of prognostic factors in three radiation therapy oncology group (RTOG) brain metastases trials. Int J Radiat Oncol Biol Phys 1997;37:745–51.
3. Sperduto PW, Berkey B, Gaspar LE, et al. A new prognostic index and comparison to three other indices for patients with brain metastases: an analysis of 1,960 patients in the RTOG database. Int J Radiat Oncol Biol Phys 2008;70:510–4.
4. Sperduto PW, Chao ST, Sneed PK, et al. Diagnosis-specific prognostic factors, indexes, and treatment outcomes for patients with newly diagnosed brain metastases: a multi-institutional analysis of 4,259 patients. Int J Radiat Oncol Biol Phys 2010;77: 655–61.
5. Markesbery WR, Brooks WH, Gupta GD, et al. Treatment for patients with cerebral metastases. Arch Neurol 1978;35:754–6.
6. Ruderman NB, Hall TC. Use of glucocorticoids in the palliative treatment of metastatic brain tumors. Cancer 1965;18:298–306.
7. Borgelt B, Gelber R, Kramer S, et al. The palliation of brain metastases: final results of the first two studies by the radiation therapy oncology group. Int J Radiat Oncol Biol Phys 1980;6:1–9.
8. Graham PH, Bucci J, Browne L. Randomized comparison of whole brain radiotherapy, 20 Gy in four daily fractions versus 40 Gy in 20 twice-daily fractions, for brain metastases. Int J Radiat Oncol Biol Phys 2010;77:648–54.
9. Murray KJ, Scott C, Greenberg HM, et al. A randomized phase III study of accelerated hyperfractionation versus standard in patients with unresected brain metastases: a report of the radiation therapy oncology group (RTOG) 9104. Int J Radiat Oncol Biol Phys 1997;39:571–4.
10. Priestman TJ, Dunn J, Brada M, et al. Final results of the Royal College of Radiologists' trial comparing two different radiotherapy schedules in the treatment of cerebral metastases. Clin Oncol (R Coll Radiol) 1996;8:308–15.
11. Phillips TL, Scott CB, Leibel SA, et al. Results of a randomized comparison of radiotherapy and bromodeoxyuridine with radiotherapy alone for brain metastases: report of RTOG trial 89–05. Int J Radiat Oncol Biol Phys 1995;33:339–48.
12. Epstein BE, Scott CB, Sause WT, et al. Improved survival duration in patients with unresected solitary brain metastasis using accelerated hyperfractionated radiation therapy at total doses of 54.4 gray and greater. Results of radiation therapy oncology group 85–28. Cancer 1993;71:1362–7.
13. Sause WT, Scott C, Krisch R, et al. Phase I/II trial of accelerated fractionation in brain metastases RTOG 85–28. Int J Radiat Oncol Biol Phys 1993;26:653–7.
14. Haie-Meder C, Pellae-Cosset B, Laplanche A, et al. Results of a randomized clinical trial comparing two radiation schedules in the palliative treatment of brain metastases. Radiother Oncol 1993;26:111–6.
15. Komarnicky LT, Phillips TL, Martz K, et al. A randomized phase III protocol for the evaluation of misonidazole combined with radiation in the treatment of patients with brain metastases (RTOG-7916). Int J Radiat Oncol Biol Phys 1991;20:53–8.
16. Hoskin PJ, Crow J, Ford HT. The influence of extent and local management on the outcome of radiotherapy for brain metastases. Int J Radiat Oncol Biol Phys 1990;19:111–5.
17. Kurtz JM, Gelber R, Brady LW, et al. The palliation of brain metastases in a favorable patient population: a randomized clinical trial by the radiation therapy oncology group. Int J Radiat Oncol Biol Phys 1981; 7:891–5.
18. Chatani M, Matayoshi Y, Masaki N, et al. Radiation therapy for brain metastases from lung carcinoma. Prospective randomized trial according to the level of lactate dehydrogenase. Strahlenther Onkol 1994;170:155–61.
19. Chatani M, Teshima T, Hata K, et al. Whole brain irradiation for metastases from lung carcinoma. A clinical investigation. Acta Radiol Oncol 1985;24: 311–4.
20. Davey P, Hoegler D, Ennis M, et al. A phase III study of accelerated versus conventional hypofractionated whole brain irradiation in patients of good performance status with brain metastases not suitable for surgical excision. Radiother Oncol 2008; 88:173–6.
21. Patchell RA, Tibbs PA, Walsh JW, et al. A randomized trial of surgery in the treatment of single metastases to the brain. N Engl J Med 1990;322:494–500.
22. Vecht CJ, Haaxma-Reiche H, Noordijk EM, et al. Treatment of single brain metastasis: radiotherapy alone or combined with neurosurgery? Ann Neurol 1993;33:583–90.
23. Mintz AH, Kestle J, Rathbone MP, et al. A randomized trial to assess the efficacy of surgery in addition to radiotherapy in patients with a single cerebral metastasis. Cancer 1996;78:1470–6.
24. Sause WT, Crowley JJ, Morantz R, et al. Solitary brain metastasis: results of an RTOG/SWOG protocol evaluation surgery + RT versus RT alone. Am J Clin Oncol 1990;13:427–32.
25. Patchell RA, Tibbs PA, Regine WF, et al. Postoperative radiotherapy in the treatment of single

metastases to the brain: a randomized trial. JAMA 1998;280:1485–9.

26. Kocher M, Mueller RP, Abacioglu MU, et al. Adjuvant whole brain radiotherapy vs. observation after radio-surgery or surgical resection of 1–3 cerebral meta-stases—results of the EORTC 22952–26001 study. Int J Radiat Oncol Biol Phys 2009;75:S5.

27. Andrews DW, Scott CB, Sperduto PW, et al. Whole brain radiation therapy with or without stereotactic radiosurgery boost for patients with one to three brain metastases: phase III results of the RTOG 9508 randomised trial. Lancet 2004;363:1665–72.

28. Kondziolka D, Patel A, Lunsford LD, et al. Stereo-tactic radiosurgery plus whole brain radiotherapy versus radiotherapy alone for patients with multiple brain metastases. Int J Radiat Oncol Biol Phys 1999;45:427–34.

29. Aoyama H, Shirato H, Tago M, et al. Stereotactic ra-diosurgery plus whole-brain radiation therapy vs stereotactic radiosurgery alone for treatment of brain metastases: a randomized controlled trial. JAMA 2006;295:2483–91.

30. Chang EL, Wefel JS, Hess KR, et al. Neurocognition in patients with brain metastases treated with radio-surgery or radiosurgery plus whole-brain irradiation: a randomised controlled trial. Lancet Oncol 2009;10: 1037–44.

31. Aoyama H, Tago M, Kato N, et al. Neurocognitive function of patients with brain metastasis who received either whole brain radiotherapy plus stereotactic radiosurgery or radiosurgery alone. Int J Radiat Oncol Biol Phys 2007;68:1388–95.

32. Li J, Bentzen SM, Renschler M, et al. Regression after whole-brain radiation therapy for brain metas-tases correlates with survival and improved neuro-cognitive function. J Clin Oncol 2007;25:1260–6.

33. Regine WF, Schmitt FA, Scott CB, et al. Feasibility of neurocognitive outcome evaluations in patients with brain metastases in a multi-institutional cooperative group setting: results of radiation therapy oncology group trial BR-0018. Int J Radiat Oncol Biol Phys 2004;58:1346–52.

34. Meyers CA, Smith JA, Bezjak A, et al. Neurocogni-tive function and progression in patients with brain metastases treated with whole-brain radiation and motexafin gadolinium: results of a randomized phase III trial. J Clin Oncol 2004;22:157–65.

35. Newcomer JW, Craft S, Hershey T, et al. Glucocorticoid-induced impairment in declarative memory perfor-mance in adult humans. J Neurosci 1994;14:2047–53.

36. Pereira J, Hanson J, Bruera E. The frequency and clinical course of cognitive impairment in patients with terminal cancer. Cancer 1997;79:835–42.

37. Mehta MP, Rodrigus P, Terhaard CH, et al. Survival and neurologic outcomes in a randomized trial of motexafin gadolinium and whole-brain radiation therapy in brain metastases. J Clin Oncol 2003;21: 2529–36.

38. Guerrieri M, Wong K, Ryan G, et al. A randomised phase III study of palliative radiation with concomi-tant carboplatin for brain metastases from non-small cell carcinoma of the lung. Lung Cancer 2004;46:107–11.

39. Ushio Y, Arita N, Hayakawa T, et al. Chemotherapy of brain metastases from lung carcinoma: a controlled randomized study. Neurosurgery 1991;28:201–5.

40. Neuhaus T, Ko Y, Muller RP, et al. A phase III trial of topotecan and whole brain radiation therapy for patients with CNS-metastases due to lung cancer. Br J Cancer 2009;100:291–7.

41. Knisely JP, Berkey B, Chakravarti A, et al. A phase III study of conventional radiation therapy plus thalido-mide versus conventional radiation therapy for multiple brain metastases (RTOG 0118). Int J Radiat Oncol Biol Phys 2008;71:79–86.

42. Gondi V, Tome WA, Marsh J, et al. Estimated risk of perihippocampal disease progression after hippo-campal avoidance during whole-brain radiotherapy: safety profile for RTOG 0933. Radiother Oncol 2010; 95(3):327–31.

Radiosurgical Management of Brain Metastases

Anthony L. D'Ambrosio, MD[a,b,c,*], Chad DeYoung, MD[d],
Steven R. Isaacson, MD[e]

KEYWORDS

- Brain • Management • Metastasis • Metastases
- Radiation • Radiosurgery

Stereotactic radiosurgery (SRS) has been established as an excellent treatment option for a large subset of patients with metastatic brain disease. Evidence-based practice guidelines have recently been published attempting to consolidate the wide variety of data available regarding when and how to implement SRS in the comprehensive treatment of this heterogeneous patient population.[1] Although class I evidence is sparse in the current literature, many effective treatment paradigms have evolved centered around SRS.

STEREOTACTIC RADIOSURGERY—OVERVIEW

SRS is a technique for treating lesions with a high dose of ionizing radiation, usually in a single session, using a stereotactic apparatus for accurate localization and patient immobilization.[2] Unlike whole-brain radiation therapy (WBRT), SRS is designed to deliver a high amount of radiation to a focal target while minimizing the dose to surrounding brain tissue.[3] The radiation dose within the target (ie, tumor) is much higher than that of surrounding tissue because of the sharp dose gradient achieved by multiple intersecting beams

of radiation.[3] Pathophysiological mechanisms behind the tumor-killing effects of SRS are not well established but likely involve endothelial cell damage, microvascular dysfunction, and the immune response.[4–7]

SRS is currently performed with 3 modalities: protons and heavier charged particles, linear accelerator–produced bremsstrahlung x-ray beams, and the ^{60}Co Leksell Gamma Unit (LGU) (**Fig. 1**).[2] Proton-beam SRS uses a cyclotron-based device capable of precisely controlling the depth of proton penetration at the target, thereby depositing most of its energy within the tumor. Few institutions use this technology because of expense and space constraints. Linear accelerators (LINAC) are used to generate a high-energy x-ray beam by accelerating an electron at a metal target. These beams are sequentially directed at the tumor from multiple static beams or arcs through multileaf collimators. LINAC technology is versatile in that it can be modified to perform a variety of radiation procedures in multiple anatomic locations and its utility is not limited to cranial applications. Gamma knife radiosurgery (GKRS) is a technology dedicated to cranial and upper head and neck disease processes. The

The authors have nothing to disclose.

[a] Department of Neurological Surgery, Columbia University College of Physicians and Surgeons, The Neurological Institute, 710 West 168th Street, 4th Floor, New York, NY 10032, USA

[b] Blumenthal Cancer Center, The Valley Hospital, 1200 East Ridgewood Avenue, Suite 200, Ridgewood, NJ 07450, USA

[c] Division of Neurological Surgery, St Joseph's Regional Medical Center, Paterson, NJ, USA

[d] Department of Radiation Oncology, The Valley Hospital, 223 North, Van Dien Avenue, Ridgewood, NJ 07450, USA

[e] Department of Radiation Oncology, Columbia University College of Physicians and Surgeons, 622 West 168th Street, New York, NY 10032, USA

* Corresponding author. Blumenthal Cancer Center, The Valley Hospital, 1200 East Ridgewood Avenue, Suite 200, Ridgewood, NJ 07450.

E-mail address: ad504@columbia.edu

Neurosurg Clin N Am 22 (2011) 45–51
doi:10.1016/j.nec.2010.08.002
1042-3680/11/$ — see front matter © 2011 Elsevier Inc. All rights reserved.

GKRS unit is composed of 192 individual ^{60}Co-based sources arranged in a conical tungsten shell designed to focus convergent gamma-ray beams at the target under control of a treatment computer. As a dedicated cranial unit, newer versions of this technology are designed to rapidly and efficiently treat multiple intracranial targets in a single planning session. Randomized trials comparing the efficacy of one SRS technology to another have not been performed. As a result, the decision to use one technology over another is subjective and based on physician preference and machine availability.[3]

CLINICAL EVIDENCE

Many questions remain unanswered in terms of the best and most appropriate treatment strategy for any one particular patient with metastatic brain

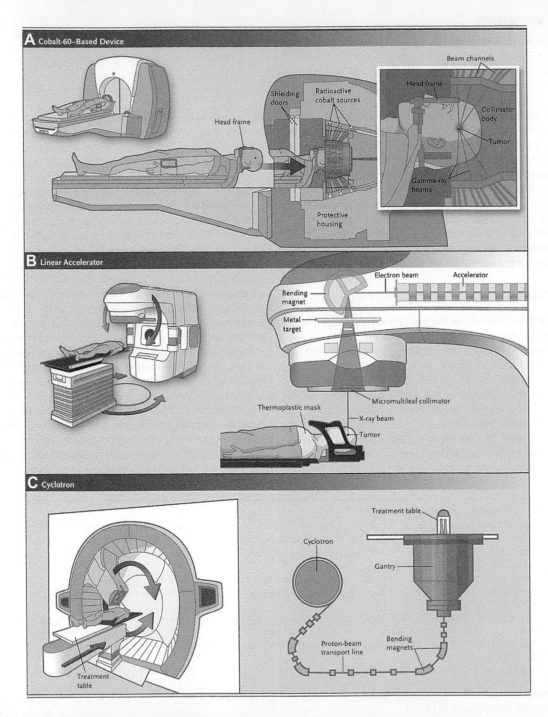

A   Cobalt-60–Based Device

Beam channels

Shielding doors

Radioactive cobalt sources

Head frame

Head frame

Collimator body

Tumor

Gamma-ray beams

Protective housing

B   Linear Accelerator

Electron beam   Accelerator

Bending magnet

Metal target

Micromultileaf collimator

Thermoplastic mask

X-ray beam

Tumor

C   Cyclotron

Treatment table

Cyclotron

Gantry

Proton-beam transport line

Bending magnets

Treatment table

disease. The overarching goals of any treatment strategy must be to maximize patient survival and quality of life while controlling central nervous system disease burden. Recently published evidenced-based practice guidelines provide an excellent review and quality assessment of the current literature regarding the role of SRS in the management of patients with metastatic brain tumors.[1] As with all complex disease processes, patients must always be treated on a case-by-case basis. In the current section, several SRS treatment combination strategies are discussed.

Stereotactic Radiosurgery and Whole-Brain Radiotherapy

Historically, WBRT has played a significant role in the treatment of patients with brain metastases. Conceptually, radiating the entire brain once a systemic cancer has demonstrated an ability to colonize and grow within the central nervous system makes sense and data have clearly supported the beneficial effects of WBRT on disease control and survival.[8] More focused radiation administration techniques, as provided by single- or multiple-fraction SRS, represent another powerful tool in the fight against brain metastases.

The literature clearly supports the finding that a combination of single-fraction SRS in addition to WBRT has superior local tumor control rates when compared with WBRT alone for patients harboring as many as 4 intracranial metastases.[9,10] In addition, there is strong evidence that combining SRS and WBRT provides a significant survival benefit for functionally independent patients with only one brain metastasis.[10] Evidence also suggests that a similar survival advantage exists for patients with multiple brain metastases; however,[11,12] prospective studies designed to specifically address this question are lacking.

Stereotactic Radiosurgery Alone

Single-fraction SRS alone has been compared with the combined technique of SRS plus WBRT as well.[13,14] The best available data demonstrate equivalent survival results between patients treated with SRS alone versus SRS plus WBRT, with a higher frequency of intracranial relapse in patients when up-front WBRT is withheld.[13] As a result, regular radiographic surveillance is strongly recommended at 2- to 3-month intervals if single-fraction SRS is used in isolation.[1]

The comparison has also been made between SRS alone versus WBRT alone. Relevant studies included patients with 1 to 3 metastases and analyzed outcomes based on validated parameters such as age, performance status, and systemic tumor burden.[12,14–16] Interestingly, in all of these reports, an overall survival benefit was reported in patients receiving SRS alone. The validity of this finding remains unclear and has yet to be studied in a randomized, prospective manner. It is possible that variables including, but not limited to, timing of systemic chemotherapy initiation or implementation of salvage surgical or radiation techniques may have influenced these results.

Stereotactic Radiosurgery and Surgical Resection

Only a few reports directly address the issue comparing the efficacy of SRS plus WBRT versus surgery plus WBRT for brain metastases.[17–19] For lesions amenable to either treatment paradigm, survival data would suggest that these strategies are comparable. Specific variables such as tumor

Fig. 1. *Panel A* depicts stereotactic radiosurgery involving a cobalt-60–based device (also called a gamma knife). A set of 192 individual cobalt-60 sources is arranged in a conical tungsten shell, with external shielding and internal channels shaped to focus radiation under the control of a treatment computer. Each cobalt-60 source emits gamma rays. The multiple gamma-ray beams converge on the tumor, resulting in the delivery of a much higher dose of radiation to the tumor mass than to the surrounding tissue. *Panel B* illustrates stereotactic radiosurgery involving a linear-accelerator–based device. A linear accelerator is used to generate a high-energy x-ray beam by accelerating an electron, which is directed at a metal target. The high-energy x-ray beams are focused by means of beam-shaping devices (micro-multileaf collimators) located at the head of the machine. Individual x-ray beams are directed at the tumor sequentially from multiple angles. As with the cobalt-60–based device, this results in the delivery of a much higher dose of radiation to the tumor mass than to the surrounding tissue. *Panel C* shows stereotactic radiosurgery by means of a cyclotron-based device that uses proton beams. The generation of a proton beam requires a cyclotron. Because such equipment is extremely expensive and requires a great deal of physical space, relatively few institutions use proton-beam–based devices for stereotactic radiosurgery. One potential advantage of such devices is that the proton beam can be precisely focused to control the depth of proton penetration. As a result, it deposits most of its energy within the tumor, with much less irradiation occurring beyond the tumor (Bragg peak effect). As with the linear-accelerator–based device, proton-beam devices can direct individual beams sequentially at the tumor from multiple angles. (*From* Suh JH. Stereotactic radiosurgery for the management of brain metastases. N Engl J Med 362:1119–27; with permission.)

size (>3 cm), tumor location (deep or eloquent cortex), and mass effect (midline shift >1 cm) should always be taken into account before initiating any treatment protocol, as these variables have not been studied extensively.

Only a few reports have attempted to compare SRS alone versus surgery plus WBRT in the setting of brain metastases.[16,20,21] When analyzed together, these studies remain relatively inconclusive regarding a significant difference in overall survival between treatment strategies.[1] SRS in lieu of resection plus WBRT is certainly a treatment option, and future trials designed to further investigate this question are eagerly awaited.

A strategy combining the strengths of surgical resection and SRS to treat all intracranial metastases up front while withholding WBRT can also be considered. A combination of focal treatment (SRS and/or resection) to all lesions with adjuvant fractionated SRS (2–5 doses) or local radiation therapy (RT) is yet another treatment paradigm currently being implemented at some cancer centers. As previously discussed, reserving WBRT for salvage therapy requires patient compliance with close radiographic surveillance and is implemented in an attempt to avoid potential cognitive impairment for young, functional patients with longer life expectancies.

NEUROCOGNITION AND STEREOTACTIC RADIOSURGERY

The etiology of neurocognitive decline often witnessed in patients with brain metastases after WBRT remains a topic of debate. In a recent prospective randomized trial by Aoyama and colleagues,[22] the Mini-Mental State Examination (MMSE) was administered to patients with 1 to 4 brain metastases receiving SRS alone, or SRS plus WBRT. The investigators concluded that, although the effects of WBRT on neurocognition may not be negligible, brain tumor control is the most important factor in stabilizing neurocognitive function.

In a more recent prospective randomized trial by Chang and colleagues,[23] 58 patients with 1 to 3 newly diagnosed brain metastases were randomly assigned to receive SRS alone or SRS plus WBRT. The primary end point of this study was neurocognitive function as assessed by a battery of tests including the Hopkins Verbal Learning Test-Revised (HVLT-R). This battery seems to be a more detailed assessment of true neurocognitive function compared with the MMSE used in the previous study. The trial was stopped prematurely by the data-monitoring committee on the basis that there was a 96% probability that patients receiving SRS plus WBRT were more likely to show a decline in learning and memory function at the 4-month follow-up time point. This occurred despite less frequent intracranial failures in this arm of the study. The investigators recommend initial treatment combining SRS alone and close radiographic follow-up for newly diagnosed patients with 1 to 3 brain metastases.

COMPLICATIONS

One of the assumed advantages of SRS over open resection is the less invasive nature of a single-session outpatient treatment versus a more invasive inpatient surgery. However, SRS does put the patient at risk for several potential complications that must be understood before designing a treatment protocol or initiating treatment.

In a recent clinical article by Williams and colleagues,[24] complications after treating 316 brain metastases with LINAC-based SRS in 273 patients harboring 1 to 2 newly diagnosed brain metastases were reviewed. The investigators reported every possible complication from the most severe to the most benign and reported a 40% overall complication rate, with new severe neurologic complications associated with 34 (11%) of 316 treated lesions. New-onset seizure was the most common complication, occurring in 41 (13%) of 316 lesions. Furthermore, most complications (74%) seemed to occur more than 30 days after SRS. Variables most strongly associated with complications after SRS include primary cancer progression and tumor location in eloquent cortex. Finally, steroid dependency occurred in association with 86 (32%) of 273 cases, with 21%, 15%, and 8% of these cases involving continuous steroid usage at 3, 6, and 12 months, respectively.

PATIENT SELECTION

Stereotactic radiosurgery should be considered in the initial design of any treatment protocol for an individual with metastatic brain disease. As with any medical or surgical intervention, the risks of treatment must be weighed against potential benefits. In patients with brain metastases, several patient-specific variables are predictive of patient outcome and serve as strong indices to guide treatment intervention.

The age of the patient must always be taken into account, as several large studies demonstrate that this variable is a strong predictor of patient outcome. The Recursive Partitioning Analysis (RPA) classification system (**Table 1**)[25,26] and the Graded Prognostic Assessment (GPA) (**Table 2**)[27–29] both

Table 1
Recursive partitioning analysis

Class I	Age <65 y, KPS ≥70, controlled primary tumor, no extracranial metastases
Class II	All patients not in Class I or III
Class III	KPS <70

Abbreviations: KPS, Karnofsky performance status.

Data from Gaspar L, Scott C, Rotman M, et al. Recursive partitioning analysis (RPA) of prognostic factors in three Radiation Therapy Oncology Group (RTOG) brain metastases trials. Int J Radiat Oncol Biol Phys 1997;37:745–51.

include age as a key prognostic variable for patients with brain metastases. In the RPA system, 65 years of age is the cut off for Class I patients, whereas in the GPA system, the age of the patient is stratified throughout the sixth decade of life.

Karnofsky Performance Status (KPS)[30] at the time of first brain metastasis diagnosis should always be assessed when considering potential treatment interventions. For a variety of reasons, KPS score continually appears in most prognostic assessment scales[25,26,31,32] because the functional status of the patient strongly predicts overall survival and must be incorporated into the design of any brain tumor treatment strategy.

Primary tumor status as well as the presence or progression of extracranial metastases must be understood in all patients with the diagnosis of brain metastases. This knowledge provides a general understanding of overall systemic tumor burden and strongly predicts overall patient survival. When the systemic tumor burden is minimal or controlled, patients often stand to benefit from aggressive treatment of central

Table 2
Graded prognostic assessment

	Score		
	0	0.5	1
Age	>60	50–59	<50
KPS	<70	70–80	90–100
Number of CNS metastases	>3	2–3	1
Extracranial metastases	Present	—	Absent

Abbreviations: CNS, central nervous system; KPS, Karnofsky performance status.

Data from Sperduto CM, Watanabe Y, Mullan J, et al. A validation study of a new prognostic index for patients with brain metastases: the graded prognostic assessment. J Neurosurg 2008;109(Suppl):87–9.

nervous system (CNS) disease. When the systemic tumor burden is significant, patients often will not survive long enough to realize the benefits of CNS tumor control and conservative or palliative treatment strategies are often selected.

Tumor-specific variables including the number of brain metastases have been incorporated into both the GPA[29] and the Score Index for Radiosurgery (SIRS)[32] to specifically address the potential to safely treat multiple lesions with SRS in a single session. The evidence indicates that patients with as many as 4 brain metastases stand to benefit from focal SRS strategies if other important variables such as age, KPS, and systemic tumor burden are taken into account.

Tumor location and size should also be analyzed before designing a particular SRS treatment plan, as larger lesions (>3 cm) with significant cystic components or severe associated vasogenic edema and mass effect may respond better to resection followed by radiation as opposed to radiation up front.

TECHNICAL CONSIDERATIONS

It has been our practice to prescribe the target dose in accordance with the suggestion of the Radiation Therapy Oncology Group (RTOG).[33] The total dose in that formulation is dependent on the size of the metastatic lesion or lesions as follows (maximum tumor diameter): smaller than 2.0 cm 24 Gy, 2.1 to 3.0 cm 18 Gy; 3.1 to 4.0 cm 15 Gy.

Target volumes and, thus, isocenter determination, is based on a contrast-enhanced CT or MRI scan with the patient's head immobilized in a stereotactic frame (CT-MRI fusion, if available, helps deal with the issue of spatial inaccuracy of MRI). Imaging studies used to deliver the actual radiosurgical treatment should be the same as those used to determine the nature, location, and size of the target lesion or lesions. The stereotactic CT or MRI slice thickness should not exceed 3 mm, whereas a slice thickness of 1 mm is most helpful for the large majority of cases. When determining the target volume, only the enhancing portion of the metastatic lesion should be included.

Doses prescribed will, to some extent, depend on the technology used, ie, LINAC or Gamma Knife. However, the dose will usually be prescribed to the isodose surface (50%–90%), which will encompass the margin of the metastasis, as defined by the imaging studies obtained specifically for the procedure. The prescription dose is then delivered to the 50% to 90% (maximum = 100%) isodose surface. This is defined as the minimum dose to the target volume. The minimum dose is established by that particular device's SRS treatment-planning software. Alternatively, the Isodose distribution on each axial level of the target and the target dose-volume histogram can be assessed. A conformality index defined as the volume of tissue receiving the prescription dose (tumor plus normal brain) divided by the volume of normal brain receiving prescription dose should be kept to less than 2.0. In other words, the volume of normal brain receiving the prescription dose should not exceed the volume of the tumor being treated.

Patients with multiple brain metastases have each lesion treated to an SRS dose level according to its maximal diameter (see earlier in this article). Some lesions may be close together, within 1 to 2 cm of each other. If possible, we agree with RTOG guidelines in trying to limit the intervening dose to 13 Gy. Individual lesion size is also an important consideration in treating multiple lesions. If one lesion is larger than 3.0 cm, treating the remaining targets has been more problematic. As the effort to treat greater numbers of metastatic lesions in the hopes of avoiding whole-brain radiation evolves, the intervening doses may not provide for the minimizing of neurocognitive toxicity gained by eliminating whole-brain radiation.

SUMMARY

SRS should be considered in the comprehensive treatment paradigm for all patients with brain metastases. This technique has proven benefits for local tumor control in individuals with as many as 4 lesions, and when combined with structured radiographic follow-up, will likely preserve a better quality of life for appropriately selected patients. Institutions and physicians treating patients with brain metastases should have the capability of safely performing SRS and individual cases should be prospectively reviewed by multidisciplinary teams to provide the best comprehensive care.

REFERENCES

1. Linskey ME, Andrews DW, Asher AL, et al. The role of stereotactic radiosurgery in the management of patients with newly diagnosed brain metastases: a systematic review and evidence-based clinical practice guideline. J Neurooncol 2010;96:45–68.
2. Verhey LJ, Chen CC, Chapman P, et al. Single-fraction stereotactic radiosurgery for intracranial targets. Neurosurg Clin N Am 2006;17:79–97, v.
3. Suh JH. Stereotactic radiosurgery for the management of brain metastases. N Engl J Med 2010;362:1119–27.
4. Fuks Z, Kolesnick R. Engaging the vascular component of the tumor response. Cancer Cell 2005;8:89–91.
5. Garcia-Barros M, Paris F, Cordon-Cardo C, et al. Tumor response to radiotherapy regulated by endothelial cell apoptosis. Science 2003;300:1155–9.
6. Lee Y, Auh SL, Wang Y, et al. Therapeutic effects of ablative radiation on local tumor require CD8+ T cells: changing strategies for cancer treatment. Blood 2009;114:589–95.
7. Szeifert GT, Massager N, DeVriendt D, et al. Observations of intracranial neoplasms treated with gamma knife radiosurgery. J Neurosurg 2002;97:623–6.
8. Gaspar LE, Mehta MP, Patchell RA, et al. The role of whole brain radiation therapy in the management of newly diagnosed brain metastases: a systematic review and evidence-based clinical practice guideline. J Neurooncol 2010;96:17–32.
9. Andrews DW, Scott CB, Sperduto PW, et al. Whole brain radiation therapy with or without stereotactic radiosurgery boost for patients with one to three brain metastases: phase III results of the RTOG 9508 randomised trial. Lancet 2004;363:1665–72.
10. Kondziolka D, Patel A, Lunsford LD, et al. Stereotactic radiosurgery plus whole brain radiotherapy versus radiotherapy alone for patients with multiple brain metastases. Int J Radiat Oncol Biol Phys 1999;45:427–34.
11. Sanghavi SN, Miranpuri SS, Chappell R, et al. Radiosurgery for patients with brain metastases: a multiinstitutional analysis, stratified by the RTOG recursive partitioning analysis method. Int J Radiat Oncol Biol Phys 2001;51:426–34.
12. Wang LG, Guo Y, Zhang X, et al. Brain metastasis: experience of the Xi-Jing hospital. Stereotact Funct Neurosurg 2002;78:70–83.
13. Aoyama H, Shirato H, Tago M, et al. Stereotactic radiosurgery plus whole-brain radiation therapy vs stereotactic radiosurgery alone for treatment of brain metastases: a randomized controlled trial. JAMA 2006;295:2483–91.
14. Li B, Yu J, Suntharalingam M, et al. Comparison of three treatment options for single brain metastasis from lung cancer. Int J Cancer 2000;90:37–45.
15. Lee YK, Park NH, Kim JW, et al. Gamma-knife radiosurgery as an optimal treatment modality for brain metastases from epithelial ovarian cancer. Gynecol Oncol 2008;108:505–9.
16. Rades D, Pluemer A, Veninga T, et al. Whole-brain radiotherapy versus stereotactic radiosurgery for patients in recursive partitioning analysis classes 1 and 2 with 1 to 3 brain metastases. Cancer 2007;110:2285–92.
17. Bindal AK, Bindal RK, Hess KR, et al. Surgery versus radiosurgery in the treatment of brain metastasis. J Neurosurg 1996;84:748–54.

18. O'Neill BP, Iturria NJ, Link MJ, et al. A comparison of surgical resection and stereotactic radiosurgery in the treatment of solitary brain metastasis. Int J Radiat Oncol Biol Phys 2003;55:1169–76.

19. Schoggl A, Kitz K, Reddy M, et al. Defining the role of stereotactic radiosurgery versus microsurgery in the treatment of single brain metastases. Acta Neurochir (Wien) 2000;142:621–6.

20. Muacevic A, Wowra B, Siefert A, et al. Microsurgery plus whole brain irradiation versus gamma knife surgery alone for treatment of single metastases to the brain: a randomized controlled multicentre phase III trial. J Neurooncol 2008;87:299–307.

21. Shinoura N, Yamada R, Okamoto K, et al. Local recurrence of metastatic brain tumor after stereotactic radiosurgery or surgery plus radiation. J Neurooncol 2002;60:71–7.

22. Aoyama H, Tago M, Kato N, et al. Neurocognitive function of patients with brain metastasis who received either whole brain radiotherapy plus stereotactic radiosurgery or radiosurgery alone. Int J Radiat Oncol Biol Phys 2007;68:1388–95.

23. Chang EL, Wefel JS, Hess KR, et al. Neurocognition in patients with brain metastases treated with radiosurgery or radiosurgery plus whole-brain irradiation: a randomised controlled trial. Lancet Oncol 2009;10:1037–44.

24. Williams BJ, Suki D, Fox BD, et al. Stereotactic radiosurgery for metastatic brain tumors: a comprehensive review of complications. J Neurosurg 2009;111:439–48.

25. Gaspar L, Scott C, Rotman M, et al. Recursive partitioning analysis (RPA) of prognostic factors in three Radiation Therapy Oncology Group (RTOG) brain metastases trials. Int J Radiat Oncol Biol Phys 1997;37:745–51.

26. Gaspar LE, Scott C, Murray K, et al. Validation of the RTOG recursive partitioning analysis (RPA) classification for brain metastases. Int J Radiat Oncol Biol Phys 2000;47:1001–6.

27. Nieder C, Molls M. Validation of graded prognostic assessment index for patients with brain metastases: in regard to Sperduto et al. (Int J Radiat Oncol Biol Phys 2008;70:510–514). Int J Radiat Oncol Biol Phys 2008;72:1619 [author reply: 1619].

28. Sperduto CM, Watanabe Y, Mullan J, et al. A validation study of a new prognostic index for patients with brain metastases: the graded prognostic assessment. J Neurosurg 2008;109(Suppl):87–9.

29. Sperduto PW, Berkey B, Gaspar LE, et al. A new prognostic index and comparison to three other indices for patients with brain metastases: an analysis of 1,960 patients in the RTOG database. Int J Radiat Oncol Biol Phys 2008;70:510–4.

30. Karnofsky DA, Burchenal JH. The clinical evaluation of chemotherapeutic agents in cancer. In: MacLeod CM, editor. Evaluation of chemotherapeutic agents. New York (NY): Columbia University Press; 1949. p. 196.

31. Lorenzoni J, Devriendt D, Massager N, et al. Radiosurgery for treatment of brain metastases: estimation of patient eligibility using three stratification systems. Int J Radiat Oncol Biol Phys 2004;60:218–24.

32. Weltman E, Salvajoli JV, Brandt RA, et al. Radiosurgery for brain metastases: a score index for predicting prognosis. Int J Radiat Oncol Biol Phys 2000;46:1155–61.

33. Shaw E, Kline R, Gillin M, et al. Radiation Therapy Oncology Group: radiosurgery quality assurance guidelines. Int J Radiat Oncol Biol Phys 1993;27:1231–9.

Surgical Management of Brain Metastases

Christopher P. Kellner, MD[a],
Anthony L. D'Ambrosio, MD[a,b,c],*

KEYWORDS

- Brain • Management • Metastasis • Metastases
- Resection • Surgery

Secondary metastases to the brain are 10 times more common than primary brain tumors, making brain metastases by far the most common intracranial tumor in adults.[1,2] The percentage of patients with systemic cancer and symptomatic brain metastases ranges from 20% to 40%, comprising a patient population of as large as a half million patients annually in the United States.[1,3] The systemic malignancies that most commonly lead to the development of metastatic brain tumors include lung, breast, kidney, colon, and melanoma. Although 80% of the time metastatic brain tumors present after the diagnosis of systemic malignancy, this may be an underestimate given that not all patients with cancer routinely undergo neurologic imaging.[4,5]

BACKGROUND AND OVERVIEW

Surgical intervention played a role in the treatment of metastatic brain tumors since Grant[6] first reported on the procedure in 1926. The morbidity and mortality of this procedure, however, was considered high and surgery was often superseded by whole-brain radiotherapy (WBRT) and corticosteroids. Improved surgical technique, developments in neuroanesthesia, and better patient selection, however, improved outcomes after surgical resection. In the 1990s, two randomized clinical trials showed that surgery for solitary metastatic lesions improves outcomes for a subset of patients with metastatic brain tumors.[7,8]

Varying levels of evidence exist for performing surgery in different patient presentations and levels of disease burden. A recent set of evidence-based guidelines was published in the January 2010 issue of *Journal of Neuro-Oncology*, compiled by a panel of doctors from the Tumor Section of the American Association of Neurologic Surgeons and the Congress of Neurologic Surgeons. These guidelines used strict methodology to report levels of evidence existing for major clinical care questions related to metastatic brain tumors and formed a useful set of recommendations.[9–11]

The major treatment options for metastatic brain tumors include surgery, WBRT, and stereotactic radiosurgery. This article outlines the clinical evidence supporting patient selection, prognostic factors, and expected outcomes in the surgical management of metastatic brain tumors.

CLINICAL EVIDENCE
Surgical Resection and WBRT

Only one randomized clinical trial compares the role of surgery and WBRT versus surgery alone for the initial management of a single metastatic brain tumor. In this trial, published in 1998 by Patchell and colleagues,[12] 95 adult patients with good preoperative neurologic function who underwent

The authors have nothing to disclose.
[a] Department of Neurological Surgery, Columbia University College of Physicians and Surgeons, The Neurological Institute, 710 West 168th Street, 4th Floor, New York, NY 10032, USA
[b] Blumenthal Cancer Center, The Valley Hospital, 1200 East Ridgewood Avenue, Suite 200, Ridgewood, NJ 07450, USA
[c] Division of Neurological Surgery, St Joseph's Regional Medical Center, Paterson, NJ, USA
* Corresponding author. Blumenthal Cancer Center, The Valley Hospital, 1200 East Ridgewood Avenue, Suite 200, Ridgewood, NJ 07450.
E-mail address: ad504@columbia.edu

Neurosurg Clin N Am 22 (2011) 53–59
doi:10.1016/j.nec.2010.08.003
1042-3680/11/$ — see front matter © 2011 Elsevier Inc. All rights reserved.

a complete resection of a single, MRI-confirmed, biopsy-proven metastatic brain tumor were randomized to postoperative WBRT or no further treatment. Patients were stratified by primary tumor and the extent of systemic disease. The primary outcome was intracranial tumor recurrence.

The trial showed that recurrence occurred significantly more frequently in the surgery-alone group (surgery alone: 32/46 [70%] vs surgery plus WBRT 9/49 [18%]; P<.001). Recurrence in the WBRT group was less common at the original tumor site and at distant sites in the brain. In addition, if recurrence did occur, the time to recurrence was longer in the WBRT group than in the surgery group at the original tumor site and at distant sites in the brain. Most importantly, mortality was decreased in the WBRT group (surgery alone: 17/39 [44%] vs surgery plus WBRT: 6/43 [14%]; P = .003). Overall survival and the duration of functional independence did not differ between groups, however. This trial played a significant role in establishing surgery as a major component of the multimodality regimen in the treatment of solitary metastatic brain tumors.

The study by Patchell and colleagues[7] was the major randomized controlled trial that established a role for surgery in the case of solitary brain lesions. In this study, the authors randomized a total of 48 patients to surgery and WBRT (25 patients) versus needle biopsy and WBRT alone (23 patients). The results showed that recurrence at the tumor site was more frequent in the WBRT alone group (12/23 [52%] vs 5/25 [20%]; P<.02); survival was longer in the surgical group, with a median of 40 weeks versus 15 weeks (P<.01); and functional independence was longer in the surgical group with a median of 38 weeks versus 8 weeks in the radiation group (P<.005). This trial clearly established a role of surgical resection in the case of solitary brain lesions.

A third randomized controlled trial examined the question of surgery and WBRT versus WBRT alone in a study involving 63 patients.[8] The outcome measures used in this trial were survival and functionally independent survival (FIS), defined as the World Health Organization performance status of less than or equal to one and neurologic function less than or equal to one. The results showed that the combined treatment or surgery with WBRT compared with WBRT alone led to longer survival (P = .04) and a longer FIS (P = .06). This study, in addition the 1990 study from Patchell and colleagues,[7] established a role for surgery in the case of solitary lesions.

In addition to these randomized controlled trials, three retrospective studies have been published addressing the same question in particular primary disease subsets.[13–15] Two of three of these studies found no significant difference among treatment groups. Skibber and colleagues,[15] however, found that median survival was longer in the surgery plus WBRT group (surgery alone: 6 months vs surgery plus WBRT: 18 months; P = .002). The level one evidence from Patchell and colleagues,[7] supported by level three evidence from Skibber and colleagues,[15] provides sufficient evidence for solid evidence-based medicine recommendations to surgically resect solitary brain metastases in good functioning patients and to follow that intervention with WBRT.[16,17]

Surgical Resection and Stereotactic Radiosurgery

One randomized controlled trial compared surgery plus WBRT versus stereotactic radiosurgery alone for the treatment of metastatic brain tumors.[18] This trial randomized 64 adult patients presenting with a single, resectable metastatic brain tumor smaller than 3 cm, good Karnofsky score, and stable systemic disease to undergo either surgical resection plus WBRT or stereotactic radiosurgery alone. The study was prematurely concluded because of poor patient accrual. No difference was seen between groups in terms of survival, death caused by neurologic disease, or freedom from local recurrence. Freedom from distant recurrence, however, was more likely in the surgery plus WBRT group (P = .04). However, this effect was lost when adjustment for the effects of salvage radiosurgery was performed. Other positive secondary outcomes included improved functional and quality of life scores at 6 weeks in the stereotactic radiosurgery group (P<.05), but this effect was lost at 6 months.

Several retrospective studies have examined the respective roles of surgery versus stereotactic radiosurgery in combination with WBRT. The two major designs for these studies have been surgery versus stereotactic radiosurgery plus WBRT, and surgery versus stereotactic radiosurgery plus WBRT versus WBRT. Nine studies have used various combinations of these two designs, and conclude in general that surgical resection may be of benefit in treating larger lesions (>3 cm) or those causing significant mass effect (>1 cm midline shift).[10] Other retrospective studies suggest that surgical resection may have a role in treating recurrence after stereotactic radiosurgery.[19,20]

Other studies have attempted to address the combined use of surgical resection followed by stereotactic radiosurgery to the resection bed in an attempt to decrease the incidence of local recurrence.[21] Further high-quality studies are needed to more clearly define the combined role of surgery and stereotactic radiosurgery in the treatment of metastatic brain tumors.

When addressing the question of whether surgery should be used for treating multiple metastatic brain lesions, no randomized controlled trials have been conducted and little evidence exists to inform clinicians in this scenario. Sawaya and colleagues[22] retrospectively matched 31 consecutive patients with new brain metastases who were treated with either radiosurgery or surgical resection at the MD Anderson Cancer Center from 1991 to 1994. Patients were matched based on Karnofsky score, time to brain metastasis, number of brain metastases, and patient age and sex. The median survivals were 16.4 and 7.5 months for the surgical and radiosurgical groups, respectively.

SURGICAL RESECTION TREATMENT PARADIGM

Surgical resection should be considered in the initial design of any treatment protocol for an individual with metastatic brain disease. As with any medical or surgical intervention, the risks of treatment must be weighed against potential benefits. In patients with brain metastases, several patient-specific variables are predictive of patient outcome and serve as strong indices to guide treatment intervention.

Patient Age

The age of the patient must always be taken into account, because several large studies show that this variable is a strong predictor of patient outcome. The recursive partitioning analysis (RPA) classification system (Table 1)[23,24] and the graded prognostic assessment (GPA) system (Table 2)[25,26] both include age as a key prognostic

index for patients with brain metastases. In the RPA system, 65 years of age is the cutoff for class I patients, whereas in the GPA system, the age of the patient is stratified throughout the sixth decade of life.[23,24,27] One large retrospective study including 1292 patients from the Netherlands in 1999 showed that age older than 70 years was an independent predictor of mortality, with a hazard ratio of one.[28] In this cohort, age was the fifth most powerful predictor of poor preoperative functional performance, little response to steroids, extensive systemic tumor activity, and three brain metastases.

Performance Status

Karnofsky performance status[29] at diagnosis of first brain metastasis should always be assessed when considering potential treatment interventions. Preoperative neurologic and cognitive function has repeatedly been shown to be one of the most important prognostic variables in the treatment of brain metastases, independent of the treatment modality. Randomized clinical trials evaluating surgery for brain metastases all restrict patient enrollment to a Karnofsky performance status of 70 or greater, which is conventionally determined to differentiate poor and good functional status.

Primary Tumor Status

In 70% of patients with at least one brain metastasis, mortality results from the clinical effects of the primary tumor.[7] Therefore, primary tumor control is a major component of determining a patient's prognosis. Three of the four major indices for determining prognosis in patients with

Table 1 Recursive partitioning analysis	
Class I	Age <65 y, KPS ≥70, controlled primary tumor, no extracranial metastases
Class II	All patients not in class I or III
Class III	KPS <70

Abbreviation: KPS, Karnofsky performance status.

Data from Gaspar L, Scott C, Rotman M, et al. Recursive partitioning analysis (RPA) of prognostic factors in three Radiation Therapy Oncology Group (RTOG) brain metastases trials. Int J Radiat Oncol Biol Phys 1997;37:745–51.

Table 2 Graded prognostic assessment			
	Score		
	0	0.5	1
Age	>60	50–59	<50
KPS	<70	70–80	90–100
Number of CNS metastases	>3	2–3	1
Extracranial metastases	Present	–	Absent

Abbreviations: KPS, Karnofsky performance status; CNS, central nervous system.

Data from Sperduto CM, Watanabe Y, Mullan J, et al. A validation study of a new prognostic index for patients with brain metastases: the Graded Prognostic Assessment. J Neurosurg 2008;109 Suppl:87–9.

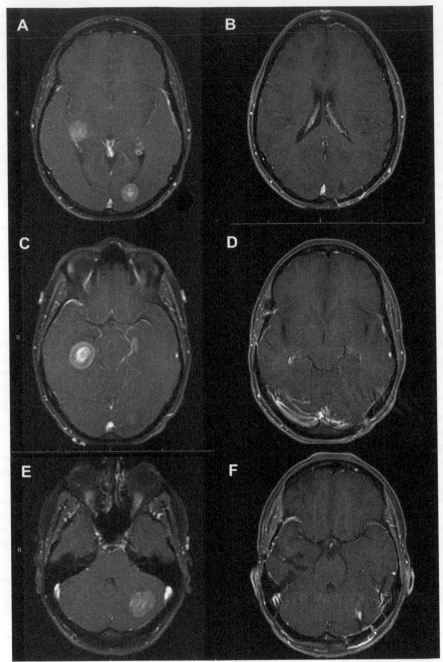

Fig. 1. T1-weighted gadolinium-enhanced magnetic resonance images depicting preoperative (*A, C, E*) and 8-month postoperative (*B, D, F*) axial images of a 29-year-old woman presenting with three metastatic breast cancer lesions. The patient's only presenting symptom was severe headaches. Karnofsky performance status at diagnosis and latest follow-up remains 100. Primary disease remains controlled with no evidence of extracranial tumor burden. The left occipital (*A*), right medial temporal (*C*), and left cerebellar (*E*) lesions were resected through three craniotomies and one surgical session. Stereotactic guidance was used intraoperatively. Postoperative radiation was administered in the form of focal fractionated tomotherapy. Each resection cavity received 4600 cGY at 200 cGy per fraction over 23 fractions. After radiation therapy, maintenance chemotherapy was reinitiated.

one to three metastatic brain tumors include primary tumor control.[25] The GPA, however, does not include primary tumor control as a major indicator. In the original article introducing the GPA, derived from the Radiation Therapy Oncology Group database, the authors justify the exclusion of tumor status from the new index by citing inconsistencies in determining the extent of primary disease caused by variability in imaging timing and type. Nonetheless, in some large database studies, primary tumor status has been shown to be one of the most significant prognostic factors, with a hazard ratio as high as 1.60.[28] Unless surgery is emergent because of severe neurologic symptoms, a full workup of the primary tumor should be completed before treatment of the metastatic brain tumor.

Status of Extracranial Disease

Several prospective databases have followed patient outcome after metastatic brain tumor resection, and recommendations have been made from these observational cohorts. The state of extracranial disease is thought to play a significant role in patient outcome independent of surgical resection, and therefore should be weighed against the probability of complications caused by surgical resection. The presence of extracranial metastases are included in the calculation of the Karnofsky performance status and the GPA.

Tumor-Specific Variables

Strong evidence shows that surgical resection of a solitary lesion is beneficial in a subset of patients. Although no high-quality studies have been undertaken to examine the benefit of resecting two or more metastatic brain tumors, some prospective studies have suggested a benefit, and therefore the consensus among surgeons has been shifting toward acceptance of multilesion resection (**Fig. 1**). Of course, the location of the lesion plays a major role in the decision to operate.

Relief of symptoms caused by mass effect or hemorrhage while minimizing neurologic complications from surgery is the goal. Lesions in or adjacent to eloquent regions are treated more conservatively. The recent development of surgical adjuncts, such as functional and intraoperative MRI, have facilitated resection of unfavorably located lesions, but no evidence yet supports their use. Histology also should be considered in the treatment plan. Hemorrhagic or radioresistant lesions, such as renal cell cancer or melanoma, also should be considered for surgical resection. Other factors that need to be considered during surgical decision making include the size of each lesion and the presence of edema.

Surgical Adjuncts and Complication Avoidance

Several surgical adjuncts recently were developed to aid in complications avoidance, particular in the removal of lesions in eloquent brain areas. Although none has been rigorously evaluated, many surgeons espouse their use and argue that they provide a strong benefit. Among these, neuronavigation has become widely popular. This technique uses pre- or intraoperative imaging to provide the operating surgeon with either a CT or MRI image of the lesion in relation to other cranial landmarks and surgical instruments.[30] Many surgeons argue that a preoperative MRI provides important information superior to a CT, such as high-resolution images of the lesion in relation to eloquent structures, surrounding edema, and lesion characteristics.[2,31,32] Functional MRI may also help in preoperative planning by showing the location of eloquent structures to avoid intraoperatively.[30,33] More recently, diffusion tensor imaging has been examined in its ability to aid in brain tumor removal with reduced complications.[33–36] This MRI imaging protocol followed the intracellular movement of water along axons, providing a view of white matter tracts and, therefore, their distortion in the presence of a metastatic brain lesion.

A new modality for potentially increasing resection percentage while minimizing complications is intraoperative imaging, such as intraoperative MRI, intraoperative CT, or ultrasound. These modalities have been poorly studied but are increasingly common. Factors preventing their current widespread use include a lack of good evidence for their ability to improve patient outcome, cost, and the loss of time necessary to conduct the imaging. Intraoperative cortical mapping may also aid in the removal of metastatic brain tumors. If the lesion is in the region of the somatosensory cortex, phase reversal of somatosensory-evoked potentials has been studied in an observational series.[37] Awake craniotomy is another commonly used and straightforward technique for intraoperatively outlining important structures.

SUMMARY

In the past 20 years, surgical resection has found an established role in the management of metastatic brain tumors. Several factors, however, make strong evidence-based medicine impossible to provide for all possible patient presentations.

These important factors, such as patient variables (eg, age, medical comorbidities, preoperative performance), tumor variables (eg, number, size, location, histology), and primary disease status must be taken into account on a case-by-case basis to guide patient selection and treatment strategy. Although progress has been made to answer some of the major questions in the management of metastatic brain tumors, several important questions remain. Future studies comparing surgery with stereotactic radiosurgery, for example, are needed to delineate patient selection, complications, and outcome for both of these important modalities.

REFERENCES

1. Shaffrey ME, Mut M, Asher AL, et al. Brain metastases. Curr Probl Surg 2004;41(8):665–741.
2. Thomas SS, Dunbar EM. Modern multidisciplinary management of brain metastases. Curr Oncol Rep 2010;12(1):34–40.
3. Society AC. Cancer facts and figures. Available at: http://www.cancer.org/docroot/stt/content/stt_1x_cancer_facts_and_figures_2008.asp. Accessed January 1, 2008.
4. Norden AD, Wen PY, Kesari S. Brain metastases. Curr Opin Neurol 2005;18(6):654–61.
5. Gavrilovic IT, Posner JB. Brain metastases: epidemiology and pathophysiology. J Neurooncol 2005; 75(1):5–14.
6. Grant FC. Concerning intracranial malignant metastases: their frequency and the value of surgery in their treatment. Ann Surg 1926;84(5):635–46.
7. Patchell RA, Tibbs PA, Walsh JW, et al. A randomized trial of surgery in the treatment of single metastases to the brain. N Engl J Med 1990;322(8):494–500.
8. Vecht CJ, Haaxma-Reiche H, Noordijk EM, et al. Treatment of single brain metastasis: radiotherapy alone or combined with neurosurgery? Ann Neurol 1993;33(6):583–90.
9. Al-Shamy G, Sawaya R. Management of brain metastases: the indispensable role of surgery. J Neurooncol 2009;92(3):275–82.
10. Weinberg JS, Lang FF, Sawaya R. Surgical management of brain metastases. Curr Oncol Rep 2001; 3(6):476–83.
11. Soffietti R, Ruda R, Trevisan E. Brain metastases: current management and new developments. Curr Opin Oncol 2008;20(6):676–84.
12. Patchell RA, Tibbs PA, Regine WF, et al. Postoperative radiotherapy in the treatment of single metastases to the brain: a randomized trial. JAMA 1998;280(17):1485–9.
13. Armstrong JG, Wronski M, Galicich J, et al. Postoperative radiation for lung cancer metastatic to the brain. J Clin Oncol 1994;12(11):2340–4.
14. Hagen NA, Cirrincione C, Thaler HT, et al. The role of radiation therapy following resection of single brain metastasis from melanoma. Neurology 1990;40(1): 158–60.
15. Skibber JM, Soong SJ, Austin L, et al. Cranial irradiation after surgical excision of brain metastases in melanoma patients. Ann Surg Oncol 1996;3(2):118–23.
16. Kalkanis SN, Kondziolka D, Gaspar LE, et al. The role of surgical resection in the management of newly diagnosed brain metastases: a systematic review and evidence-based clinical practice guideline. J Neurooncol 2010;96(1):33–43.
17. Kalkanis SN, Linskey ME. Evidence-based clinical practice parameter guidelines for the treatment of patients with metastatic brain tumors: introduction. J Neurooncol 2010;96(1):7–10.
18. Muacevic A, Wowra B, Siefert A, et al. Microsurgery plus whole brain irradiation versus Gamma Knife surgery alone for treatment of single metastases to the brain: a randomized controlled multicentre phase III trial. J Neurooncol 2008;87(3):299–307.
19. Jagannathan J, Bourne TD, Schlesinger D, et al. Clinical and pathological characteristics of brain metastasis resected after failed radiosurgery. Neurosurgery 2010;66(1):208–17.
20. Kano H, Kondziolka D, Zorro O, et al. The results of resection after stereotactic radiosurgery for brain metastases. J Neurosurg 2009;111(4):825–31.
21. Karlovits BJ, Quigley MR, Karlovits SM, et al. Stereotactic radiosurgery boost to the resection bed for oligometastatic brain disease: challenging the tradition of adjuvant whole-brain radiotherapy. Neurosurg Focus 2009;27(6):E7.
22. Sawaya R, Ligon BL, Bindal AK, et al. Surgical treatment of metastatic brain tumors. J Neurooncol 1996; 27(3):269–77.
23. Gaspar L, Scott C, Rotman M, et al. Recursive partitioning analysis (RPA) of prognostic factors in three Radiation Therapy Oncology Group (RTOG) brain metastases trials. Int J Radiat Oncol Biol Phys 1997;37(4):745–51.
24. Gaspar LE, Scott C, Murray K, et al. Validation of the RTOG recursive partitioning analysis (RPA) classification for brain metastases. Int J Radiat Oncol Biol Phys 2000;47(4):1001–6.
25. Sperduto CM, Watanabe Y, Mullan J, et al. A validation study of a new prognostic index for patients with brain metastases: the Graded Prognostic Assessment. J Neurosurg 2008;109(Suppl):87–9.
26. Sperduto PW, Berkey B, Gaspar LE, et al. A new prognostic index and comparison to three other indices for patients with brain metastases: an analysis of 1,960 patients in the RTOG database. Int J Radiat Oncol Biol Phys 2008;70(2):510–4.

27. Videtic GM, Adelstein DJ, Mekhail TM, et al. Validation of the RTOG recursive partitioning analysis (RPA) classification for small-cell lung cancer-only brain metastases. Int J Radiat Oncol Biol Phys 2007;67(1):240–3.

28. Lagerwaard FJ, Levendag PC, Nowak PJ, et al. Identification of prognostic factors in patients with brain metastases: a review of 1292 patients. Int J Radiat Oncol Biol Phys 1999;43(4):795–803.

29. Karnofsky DA, Burchenal JH. The clinical evaluation of chemotherapeutic agents in cancer. In: MacLeod CM, editor. Evaluation of chemotherapeutic agents. New York (NY): Columbia University Press; 1949. p. 196.

30. Gumprecht H, Ebel GK, Auer DP, et al. Neuronavigation and functional MRI for surgery in patients with lesion in eloquent brain areas. Minim Invasive Neurosurg Sep 2002;45(3):151–3.

31. Huang B, Liang CH, Liu HJ, et al. Low-dose contrast-enhanced magnetic resonance imaging of brain metastases at 3.0 T using high-relaxivity contrast agents. Acta Radiol 2010;51(1):78–84.

32. Senft C, Ulrich CT, Seifert V, et al. Intraoperative magnetic resonance imaging in the surgical treatment of cerebral metastases. J Surg Oncol 2010;101(5):436–41.

33. Essig M, Giesel F, Stieltjes B, et al. Functional imaging for brain tumors (perfusion, DTI and MR spectroscopy). Radiologe 2007;47(6):513–9 [in German].

34. Bae MS, Jahng GH, Ryu CW, et al. Effect of intravenous gadolinium-DTPA on diffusion tensor MR imaging for the evaluation of brain tumors. Neuroradiology 2009;51(12):793–802.

35. Price SJ, Burnet NG, Donovan T, et al. Diffusion tensor imaging of brain tumours at 3T: a potential tool for assessing white matter tract invasion? Clin Radiol 2003;58(6):455–62.

36. Wang W, Steward CE, Desmond PM. Diffusion tensor imaging in glioblastoma multiforme and brain metastases: the role of p, q, L, and fractional anisotropy. AJNR Am J Neuroradiol 2009; 30(1):203–8.

37. Tomas R, Haninec P, Houstava L. The relevance of the corticographic median nerve somatosensory evoked potentials (SEPs) phase reversal in the surgical treatment of brain tumors in central cortex. Neoplasma 2006;53(1):37–42.

Management of Skull Base Metastases

Roukoz B. Chamoun, MD[a], Franco DeMonte, MD, FRCSC[b],*

KEYWORDS
• Metastases • Skull base • Management • Outcome

Brain metastasis is a common medical problem. According to the 2008 American Cancer Society Registry, it is estimated that approximately 1.4 million Americans are diagnosed with cancer every year,[1] nearly 40% of them develop one or more brain metastasis.[2] The treatment options for these patients include surgery, whole brain radiation, stereotactic radiosurgery (SRS), and chemotherapy. Considerable efforts have been made to determine the optimal management strategy. As a result, a large number of well-designed studies have been conducted, and evidence-based clinical practice guidelines are currently available.[3–6] Skull base metastases (SBM), however, have received limited attention, undoubtedly related to the relative rarity of these lesions. The current medical literature on SBM consists of case reports and small case series. Comparative studies for different treatment options are not available, and evidence-based practice guidelines are nonexistent. Currently, management of these patients is based on the limited available data In the literature and on the clinical experience of the treating medical team.

EPIDEMIOLOGY

Autopsy series reveal a high incidence of SBM. Belal[7] found a 3% incidence of temporal bone metastases in the general population; whereas, Jung and colleagues[8] and Gloria-Cruz and colleagues[9] reported a 24% and 22.2% incidence, respectively, of temporal bone metastases in subjects with a known history of cancer. Most of these metastases are clinically silent, however, and clinical series reveal a much lower incidence of SBM. Hall and colleagues,[10] for instance, noted

only a 0.13% incidence of cranial neuropathy caused by osseous metastases in subjects with breast cancer. SBM are rare among tumors of the skull base reported in surgical series. In an article reporting the experience of George Washington University Medical Center in the surgical treatment of skull base tumors, Morita and colleagues[11] found that metastatic lesions constituted less than 5% of their subjects.

In 1981, Greenberg and colleagues[12] reported the experience of Sloan-Kettering Cancer Center in the management of SBM. Their series spanned 7 years and consisted of 43 subjects. The most common tumors found were breast cancer (17 subjects), lung cancer (6 subjects), and prostate cancer (5 subjects). In a review of the literature published in 2005 analyzing 279 cases that were identified in the English and French literature, prostate cancer was actually the most common (38%) followed by breast cancer (20%). All other pathologies constituted less than 10% each, with most of them accounting for less than 5% of the subjects.[13]

CLINICAL PRESENTATION

SBM are typically diagnosed in patients already known to have metastatic cancer. In approximately 28% of cases, these lesions can be the first sign of cancer.[13] In most cases, it is thought that these lesions spread by hematogenous dissemination. Retrograde venous seeding along the extensively interconnected midline venous system has also been postulated as a possible mechanism, mainly in the case of prostatic cancer. Malignant tumors can also reach the skull base through

a Department of Neurosurgery, Baylor College of Medicine, Houston, TX, USA
b Department of Neurosurgery, The University of Texas, M. D. Anderson Cancer Center, 1515 Holcombe Boulevard, Unit 442, Houston, TX 77030-4009, USA
* Corresponding author.
E-mail address: fdemonte@mdanderson.org

Neurosurg Clin N Am 22 (2011) 61–66
doi:10.1016/j.nec.2010.08.005
1042-3680/11/$ — see front matter © 2011 Elsevier Inc. All rights reserved.

neurosurgery.theclinics.com

direct extension of a head and neck cancer. These cases, however, do not represent true metastasis.

SBM may be asymptomatic; for example, it may be discovered incidentally on routine imaging for cancer staging or during brain imaging for head trauma. SBM should be strongly suspected, however, when patients with a known history of cancer present with cranial neuropathy or craniofacial pain. Several clinical syndromes determined by the anatomic location of the lesion have been described. In their review of the literature, Laigle-Donadey and colleagues[13] found that the parasellar and sellar syndromes were the most common (29%) followed by the gasserian ganglion (6%) and jugular foramen syndromes (3.5%). No distinct syndrome could be described in 33% of the cases.

Orbital Syndrome

The orbital syndrome is characterized by orbital or supraorbital pain, frontal headache, proptosis, diplopia, and blurred vision. On examination, there is typically periorbital swelling, tenderness, palpable mass, and decreased visual acuity (**Fig. 1**).

Sellar/Parasellar Syndrome

The parasellar syndrome is characterized by frontal and supraorbital headache, diplopia, facial

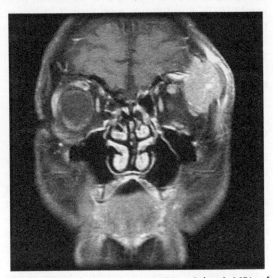

Fig. 1. Coronal, postcontrast, T1-weighted MRI of a 72-year-old man with severe pain and progressive proptosis. An orbitectomy and free-flap reconstruction was uneventful and resulted in a marked reduction in pain. The tumor was initially thought to represent a primary lacrimal carcinoma, but a small lung primary, obscured by underlying pulmonary fibrosis, was ultimately identified. (*Courtesy of* The Department of Neurosurgery, M.D. Anderson Cancer Center; with permission.)

pain, and hypoesthesia. The physical examination reveals ocular palsy, decreased facial sensation, and occasionally mild proptosis. There may be signs and symptoms of hypopituitarism, diabetes insipidus, and visual loss.

Gasserian Ganglion Syndrome

Metastases to the middle cranial base may cause pain, numbness, and paresthesia along the trigeminal nerve distribution. The symptoms can mimic those of idiopathic trigeminal neuralgia. On examination there is usually sensory loss in the distribution of one or more of the trigeminal divisions with some dysfunction of the motor root. Extension into Dorello's canal can lead to a concomitant sixth nerve palsy.

Temporal Bone Syndrome

The temporal bone syndrome is characterized by hearing loss and otalgia. Vertigo and tinnitus are much less common. The hearing loss can be conductive, related to dysfunction of the eustachian tube with secondary otitis media, or sensorineural caused by involvement of the cochlear nerve. The physical examination typically shows periauricular swelling and facial nerve palsy.

Jugular Foramen Syndrome

This syndrome is characterized by occipital or postauricular pain, hoarseness, and dysphagia. On physical examination, there is usually weakness of the palate, paralysis of the vocal cords, and weakness of the sternocleidomastoid and trapezius muscles. Occasionally, glossopharyngeal neuralgia can be part of the clinical picture.

Occipital Condyle Syndrome

The occipital condyle syndrome is characterized by occipital pain and neck stiffness. Dysarthria and dysphagia are common features of this syndrome. The physical examination typically reveals the presence of tongue weakness, atrophy, and fasciculation.

TREATMENT
Radiotherapy

Radiotherapy is currently the main form of treatment for SBM. Greenberg and colleagues[12] reported the experience of the Sloan-Kettering Cancer Center in the management of 43 subjects with SBM. All of these subjects were treated with radiotherapy. They reported an overall symptomatic improvement rate of 86%. In terms of presenting cranial nerve deficits, 16% of their subjects experienced complete resolution and 37%

experienced partial improvement. In a more recent study, McDermott and colleagues[14] reported the outcome of 15 subjects with SBM from prostate cancer treated with radiotherapy. Fourteen of their subjects showed partial or complete improvement of their cranial nerve deficits. The efficacy of radiotherapy seems to be significantly affected by the timing of the treatment. Delay in the management of these tumors results in a marked decrease in the likelihood of functional recovery. Vikram and Chu[15] found that 87% of the subjects who received radiotherapy within 1 month of the appearance of symptoms improved, compared only to 25% of those treated more than 3 months after the onset of their symptoms. In general, the authors recommend 35 Gy in 14 fractions over 3 weeks. This rapid fractionation schedule is well tolerated with little risk of long-term sequelae. For patients with controlled systemic disease and a long life expectancy, the authors recommend a more protracted course of therapy. In these situations 50 Gy at 1.8 or 2 Gy per fraction is reasonable. The authors usually cover the radiologically visible disease with a margin that includes at least a small portion of the clinically uninvolved skull base.

Chemotherapy

In addition to radiotherapy, chemotherapy, immunotherapy, and hormonal therapy are commonly prescribed based on specific tumor types. The chemotherapeutic management of skull base metastases is beyond the scope of this article.

Stereotactic Radiosurgery

Radiosurgery has been used for the primary management of skull base metastases as well as in the treatment of postsurgical or postradiotherapeutic residual or recurrence. Reported tumor control rates vary between 65% and 90%.[16–18] Iwai and Yamanaka[16] reported a series of 18 subjects treated with Gamma Knife radiosurgery. The mean follow-up was 10.5 months. In 12 subjects (67%) the tumor remained stable or decreased in size. Five subjects (28%) had complete resolution of their symptoms and 6 (33%) had a partial improvement. The main limitation of SRS is related to the size of the tumor that can be treated by this modality. Reported complication rates vary between 6% and 12%.[16,17,19] Reported complications include cranial neuropathy (optic nerve, trigeminal, facial, abducens), trismus, and cerebrospinal fluid leak.

Surgery

Recent technical advances in the surgical therapy of primary skull base tumors have made it feasible to apply such approaches to patients with a solitary metastasis. Only a minority of patients with metastasis to the skull base are considered candidates for surgical resection. These patients are critically selected based on their clinical and functional status; extent of primary and metastatic disease; pertinent radiographic studies; and the tumor's histopathology, biologic nature, and response to previous therapies. Several factors may favor surgery as a viable management option for some patients. Small cell lung cancer, breast cancer, and prostatic cancer are particularly sensitive to radiation and chemotherapy or hormonal therapy. On the other hand, melanoma, renal cell carcinomas, and most sarcomas are radioresistant and surgery should be considered. In some patients, the diagnosis can be uncertain either because patients are not known to have metastatic cancer, or because of an atypical clinical or radiological appearance of a more common tumor (eg, meningioma) (**Fig. 2**). Some patients present with rapid neurologic decline, such as visual loss, and surgical decompression can potentially improve their functional status and quality of life (**Fig. 3**).

There are few articles in the published medical literature specifically addressing this topic. Pallini and colleagues[20] reported their experience in the management of 7 subjects with clival metastases.

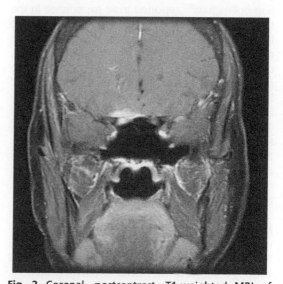

Fig. 2. Coronal, postcontrast, T1-weighted MRI of a 47-year-old woman with progressive visual decline and remote history of breast carcinoma. Imaging suggested the presence of an optic nerve sheath/anterior clinoidal meningioma. Surgical biopsy was performed for diagnostic purposes. Metastatic carcinoma of breast origin was confirmed. (*Courtesy of* The Department of Neurosurgery, M.D. Anderson Cancer Center; with permission.)

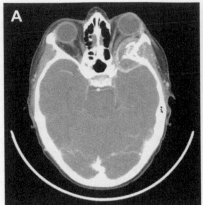 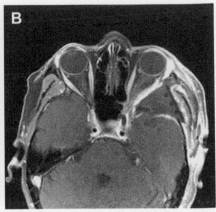

Fig. 3. (*A*) Axial, postcontrast preoperative CT scan. This 54-year-old woman with known metastatic mesenchymal chondrosarcoma presented with progressive optic neuropathy. Preoperative visual acuity was no light perception. (*B*) Axial, postcontrast, postoperative MRI. A left orbito-cranial approach was used to completely resect the metastasis to the greater sphenoid wing and decompress the left optic nerve. Vision had improved to 20/400 by the sixth postoperative day. (*Courtesy of* The Department of Neurosurgery, M.D. Anderson Cancer Center; with permission.)

The primary tumors were lung cancer (3 subjects), prostate cancer (2 subjects), melanoma (1 subject), and hepatocarcinoma (1 subject). All subjects underwent a partial resection through a transsphenoidal approach, followed by adjuvant therapy. No complications were reported. The mean survival was 12 months. The investigators did not comment on the functional outcome. Yi and colleagues[21] reported their experience in the treatment of 4 cases with metastatic tumors to the sellar and parasellar regions. A combination of approaches was used, including subtemporal, orbitozygomatic, and transsphenoidal. Two subjects had preoperative visual loss, both of them improved. One subject developed postoperative pituitary dysfunction. The mean survival was 13 months. Laigle-Donadey and colleagues[13] found the overall median survival to be 31 months. It ranged from 1.5 months and 2.5 months (for colon cancer and lung cancer, respectively) to 21 months and 60 months (for prostate cancer and breast cancer, respectively).

The authors recently reviewed the experience of M. D. Anderson Cancer Center in the surgical management of SBM (Chamoun RB, and DeMonte F, unpublished data, 2010). Between 1996 and 2009, 27 subjects with SBM underwent surgery. The most common presenting symptoms were related to cranial nerve deficits: visual loss (8), diplopia (7), hearing loss (2), facial weakness (1), and ptosis (1). Other symptoms included palpable mass (6), exophthalmos (5), headache (3), epistaxis (2), hypopituitarism (2), and diabetes insipidus (2). The median age of the subjects in this series was 52 years (14–82). Sixteen subjects

were men, and 11 were women. The histopathology of the primary tumor is summarized in **Table 1**. The most common tumors were renal cell carcinoma (6), breast cancer (3), lung cancer (2), and thyroid cancer (2). Six tumors were sarcomas including leiomyosarcoma (2), mesenchymal chondrosarcoma (1), Ewing's sarcoma (1), liposarcoma (1), malignant paraganglioma (1),

Table 1 Tumor histopathology		
Epithelial	Renal cell	6
	Breast	3
	Lung	2
	Thyroid	2
	Prostate	1
	Colorectal	1
	Melanoma	1
	Adenocarcinoma of the salivary gland	1
	Seminoma	1
	Squamous cell carcinoma	1
	Neuroendocrine carcinoma	1
Mesenchymal	Leiomyosarcoma	2
	Mesenchymal chondrosarcoma	1
	Ewing's sarcoma	1
	Paraganglioma	1
	Myxoid liposarcoma	1
	Malignant fibrous histiocytoma	1

Table 2
Anatomic location of the skull base metastasis in this series

Anterior fossa	Orbit	7
	Frontal/ethmoid sinuses	3
	Orbit and frontal/ethmoid sinuses	3
	Planum and frontal/ethmoid sinuses	1
Anterior and middle	Sphenoid wing and orbit	4
Middle fossa	Sellar/parasellar region	4
	Parasellar extending to cavernous sinus	1
	Sphenoid wing/infratemporal fossa	3
Posterior fossa	Cerebello-pontine angle	1

and malignant fibrous histiocytoma (1). The anatomic location of the metastasis is summarized in **Table 2**. Most of the tumors in this series were in the anterior cranial fossa. In 3 cases, the lesion was the first sign of cancer; whereas, in 24 cases the subjects were known to have cancer. In 18 of them the primary site of disease was adequately controlled. The SBM was the only metastasis in 11 cases. Indications for surgical resection included the need for diagnosis in 3 subjects with an unknown primary, and palliation for progressive optic neuropathy in 8 subjects, progressive proptosis/diplopia in 7 subjects, enlarging mass/solitary metastasis in 6 subjects, pain in 2 subjects, and progressive facial weakness and hearing loss in 1 subject. The most common surgical approach used was an orbito-cranial craniotomy (20 cases). The other approaches were transsphenoidal (3), transfacial (2), subtemporal (1), and retrosigmoid (1).

Seven subjects were neurologically intact; all of them remained intact after surgery. Twenty subjects had cranial nerve deficits, 7 of them improved, 11 remained unchanged, and 2 got worse (one new sixth nerve palsy and one new third nerve palsy that slowly improved over time). There was no mortality directly related to the procedure. All deaths were caused by the progression of systemic disease. A total of 21 subjects received postoperative adjuvant therapy (radiotherapy with or without chemotherapy). One subject refused radiotherapy and 5 subjects had progressive clinical deterioration caused by rapid progression of their systemic disease and the decision was to proceed with comfort care at that time. Overall, the median survival was 11.4 months. Higher Karnofsky Performance Score and absence of dural and brain invasion were associated with longer survival. Several subjects had prolonged survival. The one subject in the series with follicular carcinoma of the thyroid had no evidence of disease at the time of her death from other causes 9 years later. Patients with carcinoma of the thyroid probably represent a more favorable group in which to consider surgical resection. Effective postsurgical therapy is available with radioactive iodine and thyroid suppression. Another category of subjects that should be considered for surgical resection are those with metastatic sarcomas, especially those of low or intermediate grade. Survival has exceeded 2 years in 5 of 7 subjects (**Fig. 4**).

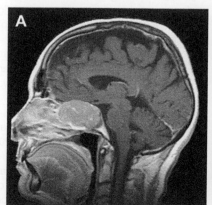 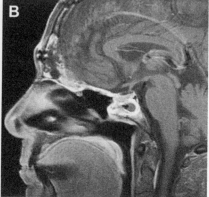

Fig. 4. Preoperative (*A*) and postoperative (*B*) sagittal postcontrast MRI of a 64-year-old woman with progressive left optic neuropathy. A bifrontal biorbital approach allowed complete tumor resection and a return to normal vision. The patient ultimately died of progressive systemic disease 26 months later. (*Courtesy of* The Department of Neurosurgery, M.D. Anderson Cancer Center; with permission.)

SUMMARY

SBM are common in autopsy studies but rare in clinical series. A high index of suspicion based on new onset cranial nerve deficit or cranio-facial pain in patients with cancer is important to facilitate an early diagnosis. The first line of treatment is radiotherapy in most cases. When administered soon after the appearance of symptoms, it can provide significant symptomatic relief. SRS is another effective form of treatment. Its main limitations are related to the size of the lesion and proximity of critical structures, such as the optic nerve. A minority of patients are selected for surgical resection. In these selected patients, surgery can provide good palliation. Ideal surgical candidates are patients with good functional status, whose systemic disease is well controlled, and who have a long expected survival. The main indications for surgery are need for diagnosis in patients with unknown primary tumors, palliation of radioresistant tumors with worsening neurologic deficit, and large solitary metastases that are accessible surgically.

REFERENCES

1. American Cancer Society 2008. Cancer facts and figures 2008. Available at: http://www.cancer.org/docroot/stt/content/stt_1x_cancer_facts_and_figures_2008.asp. Accessed May 2010.
2. Gavrilovic IT, Posner JB. Brain metastases: epidemiology and pathophysiology. J Neurooncol 2005; 75(1):5–14.
3. Gaspar LE, Mehta MP, Patchell RA, et al. The role of whole brain radiation therapy in the management of newly diagnosed brain metastases: a systematic review and evidence-based clinical practice guideline. J Neurooncol 2010;96(1):17–32.
4. Kalkanis SN, Kondziolka D, Gaspar LE, et al. The role of surgical resection in the management of newly diagnosed brain metastases: a systematic review and evidence-based clinical practice guideline. J Neurooncol 2010;96(1):33–43.
5. Linskey ME, Andrews DW, Asher AL, et al. The role of stereotactic radiosurgery in the management of patients with newly diagnosed brain metastases: a systematic review and evidence-based clinical practice guideline. J Neurooncol 2010;96(1):45–68.
6. Mehta MP, Paleologos NA, Mikkelsen T, et al. The role of chemotherapy in the management of newly diagnosed brain metastases: a systematic review and evidence-based clinical practice guideline. J Neurooncol 2010;96(1):71–83.
7. Belal A Jr. Metastatic tumours of the temporal bone. A histopathological report. J Laryngol Otol 1985; 99(9):839–46.
8. Jung TT, Jun BH, Shea D, et al. Primary and secondary tumors of the facial nerve. A temporal bone study. Arch Otolaryngol Head Neck Surg 1986;112(12):1269–73.
9. Gloria-Cruz TI, Schachern PA, Paparella MM, et al. Metastases to temporal bones from primary nonsystemic malignant neoplasms. Arch Otolaryngol Head Neck Surg 2000;126(2):209–14.
10. Hall SM, Buzdar AU, Blumenschein GR. Cranial nerve palsies in metastatic breast cancer due to osseous metastasis without intracranial involvement. Cancer 1983;52(1):180–4.
11. Morita A, Sekhar LN, Wright DC. Current concepts in the management of tumors of the skull base. Cancer Control 1998;5(2):138–49.
12. Greenberg HS, Deck MD, Vikram B, et al. Metastasis to the base of the skull: clinical findings in 43 patients. Neurology 1981;31(5):530–7.
13. Laigle-Donadey F, Taillibert S, Martin-Duverneuil N, et al. Skull-base metastases. J Neurooncol 2005; 75(1):63–9.
14. McDermott RS, Anderson PR, Greenberg RE, et al. Cranial nerve deficits in patients with metastatic prostate carcinoma: clinical features and treatment outcomes. Cancer 2004;101(7):1639–43.
15. Vikram B, Chu FC. Radiation therapy for metastases to the base of the skull. Radiology 1979;130(2): 465–8.
16. Iwai Y, Yamanaka K. Gamma Knife radiosurgery for skull base metastasis and invasion. Stereotact Funct Neurosurg 1999;72(Suppl 1):81–7.
17. Miller RC, Foote RL, Coffey RJ, et al. The role of stereotactic radiosurgery in the treatment of malignant skull base tumors. Int J Radiat Oncol Biol Phys 1997;39(5):977–81.
18. Kocher M, Voges J, Staar S, et al. Linear accelerator radiosurgery for recurrent malignant tumors of the skull base. Am J Clin Oncol 1998;21(1): 18–22.
19. Cmelak AJ, Cox RS, Adler JR, et al. Radiosurgery for skull base malignancies and nasopharyngeal carcinoma. Int J Radiat Oncol Biol Phys 1997;37(5): 997–1003.
20. Pallini R, Sabatino G, Doglietto F, et al. Clivus metastases: report of seven patients and literature review. Acta Neurochir (Wien) 2009;151(4):291–6 [discussion: 296].
21. Yi HJ, Kim CH, Bak KH, et al. Metastatic tumors in the sellar and parasellar regions: clinical review of four cases. J Korean Med Sci 2000;15(3): 363–7.

Leptomeningeal Disease

Morris D. Groves, MD, JD

KEYWORDS

- Leptomeningeal disease • Neoplastic meningitis
- Malignant meningitis • Cancer

Leptomeningeal metastasis (LMD) refers to the dissemination of cancer to the arachnoid mater, cerebrospinal fluid (CSF), and pia mater, which occurs in approximately 5% to 8% of all patients with cancer. The incidence of LMD may increase with better treatments and the overall longer survival of patients with cancer in general. The management of LMD requires the expertise of medical and neuro-oncologists, neurosurgeons, and radiation oncologists. LMD is typified by multifocal neurologic deficits and short survival in the 3- to 6-month range. The current standard of care includes external beam radiotherapy, and systemic and intrathecal (IT) chemotherapy. Future improvements in outcomes depend on: advances in the understanding of the molecular changes that allow for central nervous system seeding of cancer, the identification of subgroups of patients who can be predicted to develop LMD and in whom preventative measures can be instituted, and the development of effective drugs that penetrate, or can be directly administered into, the CSF.

EPIDEMIOLOGY

It is estimated that between 5% and 8% of patients with cancer will develop LMD.[1] Of patients with cancer who have neurologic symptoms and who undergo autopsy, as many as 19% can show evidence of leptomeningeal seeding by their cancer.[2] Based on recent data from the National Cancer Institute (NCI) Surveillance Epidemiology and End Results (SEER) Web site, the age-adjusted incidence for all cancers is 461.6 per 100,000 men and women per year.[3]

Using 300 million as the population of the United States, this equates to approximately 1.4 million cancer cases, and as many as 110,000 LMD cases, per year in the United States.

The most common cancers that result in LMD include lung cancer, breast cancer, melanoma, acute lymphoblastic leukemia (ALL), and non-Hodgkin lymphoma (NHL), but virtually any cancer can metastasize to the leptomeninges. The incidence of LMD may increase in the future because of improved survival for cancers in general. The increased use of large-molecule systemic therapies that create a sanctuary site for cancer cells behind the blood-brain barrier and blood-CSF barrier (BCSFB) may also promote the development of LMD.

PATHOPHYSIOLOGY

The seeding of cancer cells to the leptomeninges and CSF can be considered from an anatomic or from a molecular pathophysiology perspective. Anatomically, tumor cells must reach the leptomeninges to disseminate through the system. This dissemination occurs through either hematologic dissemination, via direct extension from a tumor mass adjacent to the meninges, or from a preexisting parenchymal central nervous system (CNS) metastasis[4] (synchronous or preexisting CNS metastases are found in 28%–75% of patients with LMD).[2,5–8]

Intraoperative spread of tumor cells from a CNS metastasis is uncommon but does occur as shown by the way piecemeal tumor resection (vs en bloc resection or stereotactic radiation) increases CSF dissemination rates 2.4- to 5.8-fold.[9,10] Primary

The author discloses research support from Genentech.
Department of Neuro-Oncology, The University of Texas MD Anderson Cancer Center, 1400 Holcombe, Unit 431, Houston, TX 77030, USA
E-mail address: mgroves@mdanderson.org

Neurosurg Clin N Am 22 (2011) 67–78
doi:10.1016/j.nec.2010.08.006
1042-3680/11/$ – see front matter © 2011 Elsevier Inc. All rights reserved.

CNS malignancies, such as medulloblastomas, pineal region tumors, and spinal cord tumors that reside near the CSF pathways, are particularly prone to CSF dissemination.

Once tumor cells reach the leptomeninges, they can disseminate throughout the CNS. Tumor cells can travel along the pia mater and invade the subpial parenchyma, penetrate nerves, and produce masses in the subarachnoid space. Cells can be carried in the CSF flow through the nervous system, resulting in multifocal CNS disease. The skull base and the sacral thecal sac are particularly prone to tumor cell build up because of their gravitationally dependent positions.

The molecular pathophysiology of LMD is not well understood. However, the principles that apply to metastatic disease in general[11] apply to LMD. To successfully metastasize, tumor cells must (1) possess unlimited growth potential and a high level of genomic instability; (2) be able to invade basement membranes and mobilize bone marrow constituents; (3) be able to remodel blood vessels, survive in the circulatory system and evade immune surveillance, and extravasate out of the vascular system; and (4) invade, proliferate, and establish a blood supply in the host organ.[4] These cellular activities require the hijacking of complex molecular machinery typically active during embryogenesis. Even though specific genetic mutations that produce LMD have not been identified, some molecular signals related to the disease have been found. Homing proteins, such as stromal derived factor-1 alpha[12] and angiogenesis-related molecules, such as vascular endothelial growth factor (VEGF)[12–15] are present in increased levels in the CSF of patients with LMD. These proteins may be related to the biology and development of the disease, or simply epiphenomena.

DIAGNOSIS
Clinical Findings

Symptoms and signs of LMD are related to the location of tumor deposits, or obstruction of CSF flow pathways, and are usually organized into 3 categories: cerebral, cranial nerve, and spinal.[7,8] Common cerebral symptoms and signs include headache, altered mental status, gait difficulty, nausea or vomiting, incoordination, syncope, and cerebellar signs. The most frequent cranial nerve–related symptoms are diplopia, vision loss, hearing changes, and facial weakness. Common spinal symptoms include lower motor neuron weakness, paresthesias, radicular pain, neck or back pain, and bladder or bowel

dysfunction. Multifocal symptoms and findings are typical in patients with LMD.

Imaging

Because of its higher sensitivity, gadolinium contrast-enhanced magnetic resonance imaging (MRI) of the CNS has replaced computed tomography as the imaging modality of choice in patients suspected of having LMD.[16] Imaging of the entire neuraxis is necessary to properly quantify the extent of CNS disease and to allow for a coherent and organized treatment plan. Imaging findings on MRI that are suggestive of LMD include contrast enhancement of the leptomeninges, subependyma, cranial and spinal nerves, as well as communicating hydrocephalus.[17] Typical imaging findings of LMD are depicted in **Figs. 1–4**. Neuroimaging is more likely to be abnormal in patients with LMD from solid tumors (72%–80%) versus those with LMD caused by hematologic malignancies (48%–62%).[18]

Leptomeningeal enhancement is suggestive of LMD, but not diagnostic. Therefore, one must consider other conditions that can produce similar imaging features, such as the effects of intracranial hypotension after craniotomy or lumbar puncture, as well as infectious or inflammatory diseases.

Up to 61% of patients with LMD develop CSF flow blocks at various levels along the CSF pathway.[19] Such flow blocks can result in loculation of intrathecally administered drugs, causing

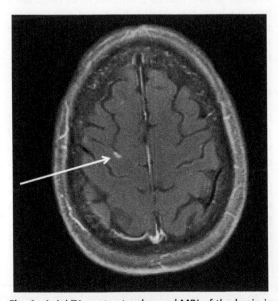

Fig. 1. Axial T1 contrast-enhanced MRI of the brain in a 44-year-old woman with metastatic melanoma and positive cytology for malignant cells. Image (*arrow*) shows subtle linear contrast enhancement along a sulcus in the right frontal lobe.

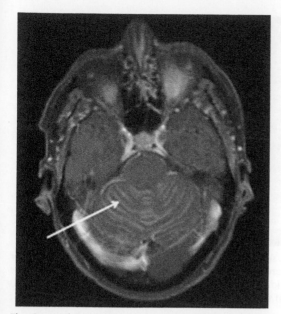

Fig. 2. Axial T1-weighted contrast-enhanced MRI of the brain in a 62-year-old woman with breast cancer and positive cytology for malignant cells. Image (*arrow*) shows prominent enhancement along the cerebellar folia, typical of LMD. This patient had a pronounced response, lasting more than 5 months, to single-agent intrathecal methotrexate.

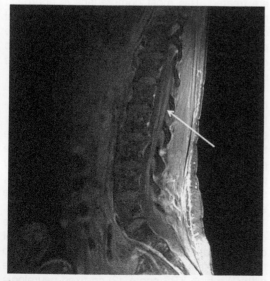

Fig. 3. Sagittal T1 contrast-enhanced MRI of the lumbosacral spine in a 50-year-old woman with breast cancer and CSF cytology positive for malignant cells. Image (*arrow*) shows shaggy contrast enhancement along the nerve roots of the cauda equina, typical of extensive LMD.

severe toxicity and impaired survival.[19] Therefore, once a decision is made to treat a patient who has LMD with intrathecal (IT) chemotherapy, CSF flow is assessed by injecting a radioactive tracer (usually pentaacetic acid labeled with indium 111). Focal radiation that opens areas of CSF flow obstruction improves survival.[19,20]

CSF

Cytologic examination of the CSF identifying malignant cells is the sine qua non of the diagnosis of LMD. However, the sensitivity of a single CSF cytologic examination can be as low as 45%,[21] and 5% of patients with LMD have normal CSF.[18] Four simple measures can increase the likelihood of finding malignant cells from a CSF sample: (1) obtain at least 10.5 mL of CSF for analysis, (2) immediately process the sample, (3) obtain CSF from a site adjacent to the affected CNS region, and (4) repeat the CSF sampling and analysis.[22] By repeating the CSF cytological analysis, one can increase the sensitivity of finding malignant cells to more than 77%.[1,8,21] Because of its higher sensitivity, lumbar space (rather than ventricular) CSF, should be used for diagnostic and treatment response purposes.[23]

Discordance between imaging and CSF findings is common. In patients with LMD who have solid tumors, CSF is negative in 17% to 23% in the face of positive MRI findings. Conversely, in patients with LMD who have liquid tumors, MRI is unrevealing in 38% to 52% of patients whose CSF contains malignant cells.[18] Because of their lack of specificity, other standard CSF analyses performed at the time of lumbar puncture can only be used to direct attention toward additional testing, rather than provide a basis for treatment. Traditional CSF analyses include CSF opening pressure, increased (>20 cm water) in 50% of patients with LMD; CSF white blood cell count, increased (>5 per mm^3) in 64% of patients with LMD; CSF protein concentration, increased (>50 mg/dL) in 59% of patients with LMD; and CSF glucose concentration, low (<40 mg/dL) in 31% of patients with LMD.[18]

To increase the yield of CSF analysis, several soluble protein and enzyme markers of LMD in the CSF have been identified.[24] Potential usefulness has been noted for CSF levels of β glucuronidase, lactate dehydrogenase, β-2-microglobulin, carcinoembryonic antigen, and β-human chorionic gonadotrophin. However, none of these molecules have become widely used, primarily because of their lack of specificity. If identified, these markers can be used to track disease progress, but the serum levels of the molecules must also be

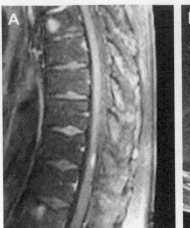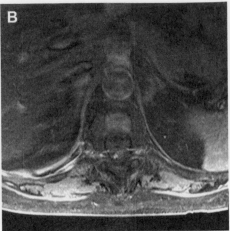

Fig. 4. (*A*) Sagittal contrast-enhanced MRI of the thoracic spine in a 64-year-old man with non–small cell cancer and malignant cells in the CSF. Image reveals an area of contrast enhancement on the surface of the midthoracic spinal cord. (*B*) Axial contrast-enhanced MRI of the thoracic spine through the area of enhancement on image (*A*) showing enhancement on the right dorsolateral surface of the spinal cord, and enhancement along the adjacent thoracic spinal nerve root.

followed to ensure that there is true CSF production rather than transfer across the BCSFB.

Recent studies have identified increased levels of molecules in the CSF of patients with LMD related to cellular homing and migration, and angiogenesis.[12–15,25,26] These may prove useful in tracking or targeting the disease, or in better understanding its biology.

In hematological malignancies, flow cytometry analysis of the CSF improves the sensitivity compared with standard CSF morphologic cytologic analysis, and is the preferred testing method when LMD is a concern.[27]

TREATMENT

Aggressive treatment of patients with LMD is controversial; this is because of the low efficacy of most treatments, the overall poor prognosis, and the risks of treatment-related toxicities. Many clinicians advise against aggressive treatment for patients with LMD. Even though neurologic deficits rarely improve, one argument in favor of treatment is that early intervention may improve quality of life and prevent neurologic death.

Treatment of LMD is considered palliative, because even aggressive treatment directed at the leptomeninges may only increase survival by 1 to 3 months.[5] Without intervention, median survival is typically 4 to 6 weeks, after which death is often caused by progressive neurologic decline.

Therapy for LMD can provide control of the meningeal disease. However, even with treatment,

one-quarter of patients with LMD die as a direct consequence of the LMD, and up to 60% die with simultaneous progression of the LMD and the systemic cancer.[28–30]

Treatment of LMD should target the entire neuraxis because tumor cells disseminate throughout the CSF pathway. For a comprehensive approach, both bulky disease and malignant cells floating in the CSF, as well as the patient's systemic disease, are treated. This most comprehensive approach requires focal (radiotherapy to bulky meningeal disease), local (IT chemotherapy for the disease present in the CSF), and systemic (systemic chemotherapy for cancer outside the nervous system) treatments.

Guidelines published by the National Comprehensive Cancer Network (2006)[31] suggest stratifying patients as either poor or good risks for survival to aid in determining how aggressive the treatment should be. These guidelines define poor-risk patients as those with (1) a low Karnofsky performance scale (KPS) score; (2) multiple, serious, fixed neurologic deficits; and (3) extensive systemic disease with few treatment options. These patients may be best served by supportive care and radiotherapy to symptomatic sites of disease. Patients who are a good risk and who may warrant more aggressive treatment are those with (1) a high KPS score, (2) no fixed neurologic deficits, (3) limited systemic disease, and (4) effective systemic treatment options.[31]

Because of physical or cognitive impairment, patients with LMD may require more assistance than is readily available. For practicality and safety, modifications of the home and special means of transportation may be necessary. Counseling to address the psychological burden of LMD on patients and their caregivers is often warranted.

Radiotherapy

External beam radiotherapy is often used in patients with LMD.[32,33] Involved field radiotherapy can be delivered to the meninges if bulky disease is present and causing symptoms (often seen with involvement of cranial nerves) or when CSF flow obstruction occurs. Thirty Gray given in 10 fractions is a typical radiation dosing scheme. Because of the higher likelihood of response, patients with breast cancer, leukemia, and lymphoma are considered best for this therapy. Even though the entire CSF system might be considered a target for radiotherapy, craniospinal radiotherapy is rarely administered because of toxicity concerns.[34]

Systemic Chemotherapy

In adults with ALL (aALL), systemic chemotherapy (SC) agents possessing high levels of CNS penetration, along with IT chemotherapy, are now standard in the prevention of LMD.[35] By incorporating CNS prophylactic regimens, the 5-year CNS relapse rate in aALL has been reduced from 58% to 8%.[35] The studies supporting the CNS prophylactic approach in adults were undertaken to try to emulate the outcomes seen in childhood ALL (cALL). In cALL, before the incorporation of CNS prophylaxis, the risk of the development of CNS

leukemia at 4 years was 75%.[36] After CNS prophylactic treatments were added, the 5-year event free survival improved to 80%.[37]

Evidence to support the use of SC (or hormonal therapy) in the treatment or prophylaxis of solid tumor LMD is less strong. However, there are reports of responses and improved survival in patients with LMD treated with SC, often without IT chemotherapy.[38–49]

Despite reports of usefulness, the use of SC in LMD is questioned because therapeutic CSF concentrations of most SCs are usually not considered to be achievable. **Table 1** lists commonly used SCs that achieve greater than 0.05 CSF/plasma ratio (a ratio <0.05 signifies nonspecific leakage of drug across the BCSFB). Reasonable approaches to treating LMD include the use of SCs with high levels of CSF penetration either with or without IT chemotherapy. However, there is a risk for increased neurotoxicity when combining such agents.[50]

Intrathecal Chemotherapy

The theory behind using IT chemotherapy is to treat (1) subclinical leptomeningeal deposits and (2) any viable tumor cells floating in the CSF to prevent further leptomeningeal seeding, thereby preserving neurologic functioning and improving survival. As noted earlier, not all clinicians advise the use of IT chemotherapy because of limited randomized data showing benefit, and concerns about toxicity.[51,52]

Table 1
CSF: plasma (or serum) drug ratios (>0.05) in rhesus monkeys or humans

Drug	CSF: Plasma Ratio	Reference
Triethylenethiophosphoramide (thiotepa)	1.0	84
Busulfan	0.95	85
Temozolomide	0.20	86
Tiazofurin	0.28	87
6-Mercaptopurine	0.27	88
5-Fluorouracil	0.155	89
Arabinosyl-5-azacytidine	0.15	90
Cytosine arabinoside	0.06–0.22	91,92
Topotecan (lactone)	0.29–0.42	93
Hydroxyurea	0.24[a]	94
Cyclophosphamide	0.20 (0.00–1.1)	95
Ifosfamide	1.2 (0.4–1.6)[b]	

[a] Oral dose of 80 mg/kg.
[b] Lowest levels in patients receiving dexamethasone.

Route of administration of intrathecal chemotherapy

To avoid frequent lumbar punctures and injury, and for possible improved efficacy of treatment, most patients with LMD have a ventricular reservoir placed for drug delivery. Delivery of chemotherapeutic drugs by lumbar puncture can result in drug placement outside the thecal sac and accompanying tissue damage. More variability of ventricular drug concentrations is seen after intralumbar drug administration. For drugs with a short half-life, intraventricular administration results in better outcomes, probably because of the more even distribution of the drug throughout the thecal sac.[53] In CNS leukemia, drug delivery via a ventricular reservoir improves the durability of remission compared with intralumbar delivery.[54] Ventricular reservoirs are usually well tolerated, but complications such as misplacement, catheter tip occlusion, and infection can occur in as many as 5% of patients.[55]

Commonly used intrathecal chemotherapies

The most commonly used IT chemotherapies for LMD from all causes include the antimetabolite, methotrexate (MTX); the pyrimidine analogue, cytarabine (Ara-C) and its longer-acting liposomal version; and the alkylator, thiotepa (triethylenethiophosphoramide). Typical schedules of administration of IT chemotherapies include a high-dose induction phase (dose based on specific drug, usually twice weekly × 4–6 weeks), followed by a less intensive consolidation phase (usually once-weekly dosing) and an even less intensive maintenance phase.[56] Dosing schemes using a concentration-times-time technique, prolonging tumor cell drug exposure, may improve outcomes.[56]

Few randomized data exist comparing the efficacy of these drugs. In the randomized studies that do exist, nonsignificant differences in survival have been shown when comparing IT chemotherapies with each other or in various combinations.[57–60] However, in lymphomatous meningitis, liposomal Ara-C results in a higher degree of tumor cell clearance from the CSF and a longer median time to neurologic progression and survival duration compared with the standard formulation of Ara-C.[61] The benefits of liposomal Ara-C seen in patients with lymphomatous meningitis were not seen in patients with LMD who had solid tumors.

ADVERSE EFFECTS OF THERAPY

Significant toxicities can occur in conjunction with the delivery of IT chemotherapy or radiotherapy to the CNS.[55] IT Ara-C can cause neuropathy, cerebellar, or spinal cord injury. IT MTX can cause acute arachnoiditis, nausea, vomiting, and mental status change and may be associated with seizures.[62] IT MTX can also cause mucositis and myelosuppression if not followed by systemic administration of folinic acid. IT thiotepa toxicity is similar to that of IT MTX; however, it may cause more hematologic toxicity.[63]

Radiotherapy can worsen myelosuppression in heavily pretreated patients who have cancer, and may raise the chance of neurotoxicity from IT chemotherapy.[64] Necrotizing leukoencephalopathy, especially when IT MTX is administered after radiotherapy, is a severe complication to be avoided. A less fulminate leukoencephalopathy, manifested by dementia, seizure, progressive tetraparesis, and change in white matter, may be more likely to occur in patients receiving IT chemotherapy versus those receiving SC.[51]

CSF flow obstruction caused by arachnoid granulation blockade by cellular debris can cause symptoms of cerebral hypoperfusion. These symptoms may be caused by a relative increase in intracranial pressure compared with systemic blood pressure and can be misdiagnosed as syncope or seizure activity. Resolution of symptoms with CSF drainage can help alleviate the patient's symptoms. Long-term management of this problem can be accomplished with CSF diversion, or through administration of acetazolamide.

PROGNOSIS

Without LMD-directed therapy, patients have survivals in the 3- to 6-week range. Death is often caused by progressive neurologic dysfunction.[5,8] Treating solid tumor LMD stabilizes neurologic symptoms in 45% of patients,[8] but even with aggressive, multimodal therapy, typical LMD survivals are in the 8- to 16-week range.[65] Patients with hematologic malignancies and LMD have better survivals (4.7 months) compared with those with LMD from solid tumors (2.3 months) ($P = .0006$).[18] Among solid tumors, patients who have breast cancer with LMD who receive treatment tend to have the best outcomes, with median survivals of 4.5 months and up to 25% 1-year survival.[6] Treatment that clears malignant cells from the CSF may correspond with improved quality of life and better overall survival.[39,58,61]

EXPERIMENTAL THERAPIES

Experimental therapies for LMD include both systemic and IT agents. None have yet shown enough promise, or are far enough along in development, to have supplanted the older interventions.

Systemic Therapies

Bevacizumab

Bevacizumab is a systemically administered monoclonal antibody targeting the proangiogenic protein, VEGF-A. It is approved by the US Food and Drug Administration for use in several malignant diseases. Recent reports found increased VEGF-A levels in the CSF of patients with LMD with solid tumors [12,13,15]; further, CSF VEGF-A levels decrease and correlate with CSF responses.[13] Similar to other large molecules, bevacizumab probably does not penetrate the intact CNS or CSF to any significant degree.[66] Systemically administered bevacizumab is currently being tested in patients with LMD with solid tumors.

Gefitinib

Gefitinib is a small-molecule tyrosine kinase inhibitor with activity against lung cancers possessing activating mutations of the epidermal growth factor receptor (EGFR). Case reports show responses to EGFR inhibitors in patients with LMD caused by non–small cell lung cancer (NSCLC).[67–69] High-dose gefitinib (5 times standard doses) was recently prospectively evaluated in patients with LMD caused by NSCLC whose tumors possess activating EGFR mutations. Early reports of the clinical outcomes are promising; final results are pending (D. Jackman, MD, Boston, MA, personal communication, June 2009).

Pemetrexed

Pemetrexed (PMX) is an antimetabolite, similar to MTX, and is approved for mesothelioma and NSCLC. PMX is active in some MTX-resistant malignancies. The CSF pharmacokinetics of systemically administered PMX are currently being evaluated in patients with LMD. The drug is unique in that it acts through several enzyme systems involved in folate metabolism and gains intracellular access through at least 4 mechanisms, possibly increasing its activity compared with MTX. There are early CSF responses in patients with LMD with breast cancer (J. Raizer, MD, Chicago, IL, personal communication, June 2009).

Intrathecal Therapies

Cytotoxic therapies

The search for more effective, less toxic IT cytotoxic therapies is ongoing. Recently tested IT cytotoxic chemotherapies with some degree of efficacy and modest toxicity are presented in **Table 2**. Of these, the topoisomerase inhibitors

seem particularly promising for further study (possibly in combination with other IT agents or systemic treatments), in light of their mild toxicity profile, and reasonable efficacy.[70,71] To try to further enhance its activity by prolonging tumor cell exposure to drug, a concentration-times-time study of IT topotecan is ongoing within the Pediatric Brain Tumor Consortium.

IT delivery of the β emitter, ^{131}I, has shown some activity in LMD. IT administration of the nonbound formulation of ^{131}I, sodium iodide, resulted in almost no toxicity and achieved CSF tumor cell clearance in 29% of patients.[72] Further testing of this agent is planned. [131]I bound to the GD2-targeted monoclonal antibody ([131]I-3F8) is being tested in phase 2 studies.[73] Phase 1 data suggest possible efficacy in childhood primitive neuroectodermal tumors and neuroblastoma.

Monoclonal Antibodies

Rituximab

Rituximab is a humanized monoclonal antibody targeting the CD-20 antigen, which is expressed on most B-cell lymphomas and leukemias. In 1997, Rituximab was approved for intravenous use in B-cell lymphoma. Because of its large size (146 kDa), the CSF/serum ratio of this molecule is only 0.001 after intravenous administration.[74]

A recently reported phase 1 study of IT rituximab in adults identified 25 mg twice weekly (9 doses total) as the maximum tolerated dose. The estimated half-life of the drug was 34.9 hours. Cytologic responses (including complete responses) and improvements in intraocular and intraparenchymal lymphoma were seen in most patients. Toxicities were mild and included chills and hypertension.[75] A smaller dose (10 mg weekly) of IT rituximab has been tested in children with B-cell ALL. In 5 of the 7 subjects, a complete response was achieved. The 2 that relapsed did so outside the CNS.[76] Further refinement of the use of this agent in applicable diseases warrants study.

Trastuzumab

Thirty percent of primary breast cancers overexpress the EGFR 2 protein (HER2), which is targeted by the humanized monoclonal antibody, trastuzumab. Trastuzumab destroys tumor cells through antibody-dependent mechanisms; it does not reach the CSF in significant concentrations, even after CNS-directed radiotherapy for LMD.[77]

Several case reports using IT trastuzumab in patients with HER2-overexpressing breast cancers with LMD showed efficacy.[78–80] Based on these findings, results from a pilot study using IT trastuzumab in patients with LMD caused by

Table 2
Newer intrathecal cytotoxic chemotherapies

Agent/N (Number of Patients)	Induction IT Dose and Frequency	Toxicity	Efficacy	Reference
Etoposide				
N = 27	0.5 mg daily × 5, every other week × 8 wk	18% mild arachnoiditis	26% CSF clearance 4% 1-y survival	70
Topotecan				
N = 62	0.4 mg twice weekly × 6 wk	32% mild arachnoiditis	21% CSF clearance 15-wk median survival	71
Mafosfamide				
#1: N = 30	#1: 5 mg twice weekly × 4 wk	#1: headache and neck pain	#1: 43% response or SD	96
#2: N = 25[a]	#2: 14 mg twice weekly × 6 wk	#2: mild irritability all patients		97
Busulfan				
#1: 28 children	13 mg twice weekly × 2 wk	#1: myelosuppression, GI symptoms common	#1: 39% SD at 2 wk	98
#2: 20 adults			#2: 30% response or SD	99
5-Fluoro-2'-deoxyuridine N = 25	1.0 mg/d continuous infusion until progression	20% bacterial meningitis	16% CSF clearance 8.4 months median survival	100

Abbreviations: GI, gastrointestinal; SD, stable disease.
  [a] Children with embryonal tumors.
  Data from Groves MD. Leptomeningeal metastases: still a challenge. Am Soc Clin Oncol Ed Book 2008:80–87.

breast cancer, medulloblastoma, or glioblastoma were recently presented.[81] IT trastuzumab was administered at 20 to 60 mg per dose, either weekly or every other week for 4 treatments, then continued every other week until progression. Responses were seen in 7 of 11 patients with glioblastoma, 2 of 4 patients with breast cancer and in the single patient with medulloblastoma. The HER2 receptor status was predictive of response. No adverse events were reported. Further study of IT trastuzumab, either alone or in combination with other approaches, is warranted.

Combination Therapies

Combination of IT and systemic therapies may improve outcomes in LMD.[42,48] Ongoing studies that combine IT and systemic therapies include a study evaluating IT liposomal Ara-C plus systemic bevacizumab in patients with LMD with primary brain tumors, and a study of oral capecitabine plus liposomal Ara-C in patients who have breast cancer with LMD (Ricardo Soffietti, MD, Turin, Italy, personal communication, May, 2010).

FUTURE DIRECTIONS

The gains seen in preventing CNS disease in cALL[82] and lymphoma[83] inspire the hope of similar advances in other forms of LMD. Similar approaches will become feasible when biomarkers with a high enough positive predictive value can be identified. Useful biomarkers could include (1) molecular changes within the primary or metastatic tumors that predict CNS or CSF metastases, (2) changes within the host genome that predict CNS and CSF metastasis development, (3) plasma or CSF biomarkers that predict LMD before its clinical development. Preliminary data suggest that CSF VEGF may be such a marker,[12] but further validation is needed. In conjunction with an effective biomarker, an intervention with a high therapeutic index will be needed.

Clinical scenarios (surrogates for the underlying disease biology) can identify patients at higher risk of LMD, and can possibly serve as signals for treatment. Recent work has shown that patients with brain metastases (BM) who undergo piecemeal resection of their tumors (compared with en bloc resection or stereotactic radiosurgery [SRS]) have an increased risk of developing LMD.[9,10] Risk of LMD in patients having piecemeal resection may be as much as 2.45 to 5.8 times higher than in those only receiving SRS. Patients with BM who undergo piecemeal resection of their tumors may be a good population in which to test prophylactic interventions against LMD.

SUMMARY

LMD is a lethal complication caused by a variety of cancers, typically developing late in the disease course. It is associated with major neurologic disabilities and short survival. The incidence of LMD may increase because of longer survival of patients who have cancer, and because of the use of newer large-molecule therapies with poor CNS penetration. The molecular changes responsible for the development of LMD are still mostly unknown.

To achieve improved outcomes for patients who have LMD, new treatments need to reach the meninges and CSF and interact with relevant molecular targets. Some of the agents currently in testing may contribute to this goal. To allow for better outcomes through earlier treatment, and ultimately prevention of LMD, stepwise advances in diagnosis are needed. These steps include the appreciation of clinical scenarios predisposing to the development of LMD, the validation of circulating plasma and CSF cellular and soluble biomarkers, and, ultimately, biomarkers derived from the genome of the tumor and host. At each step, and with agents with higher therapeutic indices, it should be possible to develop interventions based on likelihood ratios to allow for gradual improvements in outcomes for patients suffering from this devastating disease.

REFERENCES

1. DeAngelis LM, Posner JB. Neurologic complications of cancer. (Contemporary neurology series). New York: Oxford University Press; 2009.
2. Glass JP, Melamed MF, Chernik NL, et al. Malignant cells in cerebrospinal fluid (CSF): the meaning of a positive CSF cytology. Neurology 1979;29(10):1369–75.
3. Altekruse SF, Kosary CL, Krapcho M, et al. SEER Cancer Statistics Review, 1975–2007. Bethesda (MD): National Cancer Institute; 2010.
4. Groves MD. The pathogenesis of neoplastic meningitis. Curr Oncol Rep 2003;5(1):15–23.
5. Balm M, Hammack J. Leptomeningeal carcinomatosis. Presenting features and prognostic factors. Arch Neurol 1996;53(7):626–32.
6. Gauthier H, Guilhaume MN, Bidard FC, et al, Survival of breast cancer patients with meningeal carcinomatosis. Ann Oncol, April 29, 2010. [Online].
7. Harstad L, Hess KR, Groves MD. Prognostic factors and outcomes in patients with leptomeningeal melanomatosis. Neuro Oncol 2008;10(6):1010–8.
8. Wasserstrom WR, Glass JP, Posner JB. Diagnosis and treatment of leptomeningeal metastases from solid tumors: experience with 90 patients. Cancer 1982;49(4):759–72.
9. Suki D, Abouassi H, Patel AJ, et al. Comparative risk of leptomeningeal disease after resection or stereotactic radiosurgery for solid tumor metastasis to the posterior fossa. J Neurosurg 2008;108(2):248–57.
10. Suki D, Hatiboglu MA, Patel AJ, et al. Comparative risk of leptomeningeal dissemination of cancer after surgery or stereotactic radiosurgery for a single supratentorial solid tumor metastasis. Neurosurgery 2009;64(4):664–74.
11. Chiang AC, Massague J. Molecular basis of metastasis. N Engl J Med 2008;359(26):2814–23.
12. Groves MD, Hess KR, Puduvalli VK, et al. Biomarkers of disease: cerebrospinal fluid vascular endothelial growth factor (VEGF) and stromal cell derived factor (SDF)-1 levels in patients with neoplastic meningitis (NM) due to breast cancer, lung cancer and melanoma. J Neurooncol 2009;92(2):229–34.
13. Herrlinger U, Wiendl H, Renninger M, et al. Vascular endothelial growth factor (VEGF) in leptomeningeal metastasis: diagnostic and prognostic value. Br J Cancer 2004;91(2):219–24.
14. Reijneveld JC, Brandsma D, Boogerd W, et al. CSF levels of angiogenesis-related proteins in patients with leptomeningeal metastases. Neurology 2005;65(7):1120–2.
15. Stockhammer GF, Poewe WF, Burgstaller SF, et al. Vascular endothelial growth factor in CSF: a biological marker for carcinomatous meningitis. Neurology 2000;54(8):1670–6.
16. Chamberlain MC, Sandy AD, Press GA. Leptomeningeal metastasis: a comparison of gadolinium-enhanced MR and contrast-enhanced CT of the brain. Neurology 1990;40(3 Pt 1):435–8.
17. Freilich RJ, Krol G, DeAngelis LM. Neuroimaging and cerebrospinal fluid cytology in the diagnosis of leptomeningeal metastasis. Ann Neurol 1995;38(1):51–7.
18. Clarke JL, Perez HR, Jacks LM, et al. Leptomeningeal metastases in the MRI era. Neurology 2010;74(18):1449–54.
19. Glantz MJ, Hall WA, Cole BF, et al. Diagnosis, management, and survival of patients with leptomeningeal cancer based on cerebrospinal fluid-flow status. Cancer 1995;75(12):2919–31.

20. Chamberlain MC, Kormanik P, Jaeckle KA, et al. 111Indium-diethylenetriamine pentaacetic acid CSF flow studies predict distribution of intrathecally administered chemotherapy and outcome in patients with leptomeningeal metastases. Neurology 1999;52(1):216–7.

21. Olson ME, Chernik NL, Posner JB. Infiltration of the leptomeninges by systemic cancer. A clinical and pathologic study. Arch Neurol 1974;30(2): 122–37.

22. Glantz MJ, Cole BF, Glantz LK, et al. Cerebrospinal fluid cytology in patients with cancer: minimizing false-negative results. Cancer 1998;82(4):733–9.

23. Gaynon PS. Primary treatment of childhood acute lymphoblastic leukemia of non-T cell lineage (including infants). Hematol Oncol Clin North Am 1990;4(5):915–36.

24. Walbert T, Groves MD. Known and emerging biomarkers of leptomeningeal metastasis and its response to treatment. Future Oncol 2010;6(2): 287–97.

25. Corsini E, Bernardi G, Gaviani P, et al. Intrathecal synthesis of tumor markers is a highly sensitive test in the diagnosis of leptomeningeal metastasis from solid cancers. Clin Chem Lab Med 2009; 47(7):874–9.

26. van de Langerijt B, Gijtenbeek JM, de Reus HP, et al. CSF levels of growth factors and plasminogen activators in leptomeningeal metastases. Neurology 2006;67(1):114–9.

27. Hegde U, Filie A, Little RF, et al. High incidence of occult leptomeningeal disease detected by flow cytometry in newly diagnosed aggressive B-cell lymphomas at risk for central nervous system involvement: the role of flow cytometry versus cytology. Blood 2005;105(2):496–502.

28. Chamberlain MC, Kormanik P. Carcinoma meningitis secondary to non-small cell lung cancer: combined modality therapy. Arch Neurol 1998; 55(4):506–12.

29. Chamberlain MC, Kormanik PR. Carcinomatous meningitis secondary to breast cancer: predictors of response to combined modality therapy. J Neurooncol 1997;35(1):55–64.

30. Jaeckle KA, Phuphanich S, Bent MJ, et al. Intrathecal treatment of neoplastic meningitis due to breast cancer with a slow-release formulation of cytarabine. Br J Cancer 2001;84(2):157–63.

31. Grossman SA, Spence A. NCCN clinical practice guidelines for carcinomatous/lymphomatous meningitis. Oncology 1999;13(11A):144–52.

32. Chang EL, Maor MH. Standard and novel radiotherapeutic approaches to neoplastic meningitis. Curr Oncol Rep 2003;5(1):24–8.

33. Feyer P, Sautter-Bihl ML, Budach W, et al. DEGRO Practical Guidelines for palliative radiotherapy of breast cancer patients: brain metastases and leptomeningeal carcinomatosis. Strahlenther Onkol 2010;186(2):63–9.

34. Chamberlain MC. Neoplastic meningitis. Oncologist 2008;13(9):967–77.

35. Cortes J, O'Brien SM, Pierce S, et al. The value of high-dose systemic chemotherapy and intrathecal therapy for central nervous system prophylaxis in different risk groups of adult acute lymphoblastic leukemia. Blood 1995;86(6):2091–7.

36. Evans AE, Gilbert ES, Zandstra R. The increasing incidence of central nervous system leukemia in children. (Children's Cancer Study Group A). Cancer 1970;26(2):404–9.

37. Smith M, Arthur D, Camitta B, et al. Uniform approach to risk classification and treatment assignment for children with acute lymphoblastic leukemia. J Clin Oncol 1996;14(1):18–24.

38. Boogerd W, Dorresteijn LD, van Der S, et al. Response of leptomeningeal metastases from breast cancer to hormonal therapy. Neurology 2000;55(1):117–9.

39. Boogerd W, Hart AA, van der Sande JJ, et al. Meningeal carcinomatosis in breast cancer. Prognostic factors and influence of treatment. Cancer 1991;67(6):1685–95.

40. Boogerd W, van den Bent MJ, Koehler PJ, et al. The relevance of intraventricular chemotherapy for leptomeningeal metastasis in breast cancer: a randomised study. Eur J Cancer 2004;40(18):2726–33.

41. de Wit M, Lange-Brock V, Kruell A, et al. Leptomeningeal metastases: results of different therapeutic approaches. J Clin Oncol 2007;25(18).

42. Fizazi K, Asselain B, Vincent-Salomon A, et al. Meningeal carcinomatosis in patients with breast carcinoma. Clinical features, prognostic factors, and results of a high-dose intrathecal methotrexate regimen. Cancer 1996;77(7):1315–23.

43. Giglio P, Tremont-Lukats IW, Groves MD. Response of neoplastic meningitis from solid tumors to oral capecitabine. J Neurooncol 2003;65(2):167–72.

44. Grant R, Naylor B, Greenberg HS, et al. Clinical outcome in aggressively treated meningeal carcinomatosis. Arch Neurol 1994;51(5):457–61.

45. Herrlinger U, Forschler H, Kuker W, et al. Leptomeningeal metastasis: survival and prognostic factors in 155 patients. J Neurol Sci 2004;223(2):167–78.

46. Mencel PJ, DeAngelis LM, Motzer RJ. Hormonal ablation as effective therapy for carcinomatous meningitis from prostatic carcinoma. Cancer 1994;73(7):1892–4.

47. Ozdogan M, Samur M, Bozcuk HS, et al. Durable remission of leptomeningeal metastasis of breast cancer with letrozole: a case report and implications of biomarkers on treatment selection. Jpn J Clin Oncol 2003;33(5):229–31.

48. Rudnicka H, Niwinska A, Murawska M. Breast cancer leptomeningeal metastasis—the role of

multimodality treatment. J Neurooncol 2007;84(1): 57–62.

49. Siegal T, Lossos A, Pfeffer MR. Leptomeningeal metastases: analysis of 31 patients with sustained off-therapy response following combined-modality therapy. Neurology 1994;44(8):1463–9.

50. Jabbour E, O'Brien S, Kantarjian H, et al. Neurologic complications associated with intrathecal liposomal cytarabine given prophylactically in combination with high-dose methotrexate and cytarabine to patients with acute lymphocytic leukemia. Blood 2007;109(8):3214–8.

51. Bokstein F, Lossos A, Siegal T. Leptomeningeal metastases from solid tumors: a comparison of two prospective series treated with and without intra-cerebrospinal fluid chemotherapy. Cancer 1998;82(9):1756–63.

52. Glantz MJ, Cole BF, Recht L, et al. High-dose intravenous methotrexate for patients with nonleukemic leptomeningeal cancer: is intrathecal chemotherapy necessary? J Clin Oncol 1998;16(4):1561–7.

53. Glantz MJ, Van HA, Fisher R, et al. Route of intracerebrospinal fluid chemotherapy administration and efficacy of therapy in neoplastic meningitis. Cancer 2010;116(8):1947–52.

54. Bleyer WA, Poplack DG. Intraventricular versus intralumbar methotrexate for central-nervous-system leukemia: prolonged remission with the Ommaya reservoir. Med Pediatr Oncol 1979;6(3):207–13.

55. Chamberlain MC, Kormanik PA, Barba D. Complications associated with intraventricular chemotherapy in patients with leptomeningeal metastases. J Neurosurg 1997;87(5):694–9.

56. Chamberlain MC. Neoplastic meningitis. Neurologist 2006;12(4):179–87.

57. Glantz MJ, Jaeckle KA, Chamberlain MC, et al. A randomized controlled trial comparing intrathecal sustained-release cytarabine (DepoCyt) to intrathecal methotrexate in patients with neoplastic meningitis from solid tumors. Clin Cancer Res 1999;5(11):3394–402.

58. Hitchins RN, Bell DR, Woods RL, et al. A prospective randomized trial of single-agent versus combination chemotherapy in meningeal carcinomatosis. J Clin Oncol 1987;5(10):1655–62.

59. Shapiro WR, Schmid M, Glantz M, et al. A randomized phase III/IV study to determine benefit and safety of cytarabine liposome injection for treatment of neoplastic meningitis. Proceedings of the American Society of Clinical Oncology 2006; 24(18).

60. Trump DL, Grossman SA, Thompson G, et al. Treatment of neoplastic meningitis with intraventricular thiotepa and methotrexate. Cancer Treat Rep 1982;66(7):1549–51.

61. Glantz MJ, LaFollette S, Jaeckle KA, et al. Randomized trial of a slow-release versus a standard formulation of cytarabine for the intrathecal treatment of lymphomatous meningitis. J Clin Oncol 1999;17(10):3110–6.

62. Bleyer WA, Drake JC, Chabner BA. Neurotoxicity and elevated cerebrospinal-fluid methotrexate concentration in meningeal leukemia. N Engl J Med 1973;289(15):770–3.

63. Grossman SA, Finkelstein DM, Ruckdeschel JC, et al. Randomized prospective comparison of intraventricular methotrexate and thiotepa in patients with previously untreated neoplastic meningitis. Eastern Cooperative Oncology Group. J Clin Oncol 1993;11(3):561–9.

64. Bleyer WA. Neurologic sequelae of methotrexate and ionizing radiation: a new classification. Cancer Treat Rep 1981;65(Suppl 1):89–98.

65. Groves MD. Leptomeningeal carcinomatosis: diagnosis and management. In: Sawaya R, editor. Intracranial metastases: current management strategies. Malden (MA): Blackwell Futura; 2004. p. 309–30.

66. Pestalozzi BC, Brignoli S. Trastuzumab in CSF. J Clin Oncol 2000;18(11):2349–51.

67. Choong NW, Dietrich S, Seiwert TY, et al. Gefitinib response of erlotinib-refractory lung cancer involving meninges—role of EGFR mutation. Nat Clin Pract Oncol 2006;3(1):50–7.

68. Jackman DM, Holmes AJ, Lindeman N, et al. Response and resistance in a non-small-cell lung cancer patient with an epidermal growth factor receptor mutation and leptomeningeal metastases treated with high-dose gefitinib. J Clin Oncol 2006;24(27):4517–20.

69. Kanaji N, Bandoh S, Nagamura N, et al. Significance of an epidermal growth factor receptor mutation in cerebrospinal fluid for carcinomatous meningitis. Intern Med 2007;46(19):1651–5.

70. Chamberlain MC, Tsao-Wei DD, Groshen S. Phase II trial of intracerebrospinal fluid etoposide in the treatment of neoplastic meningitis. Cancer 2006; 106(9):2021–7.

71. Groves MD, Glantz MJ, Chamberlain MC, et al. A multicenter phase II trial of intrathecal topotecan in patients with meningeal malignancies. Neuro Oncol 2008;10(2):208–15.

72. Wong FC, Groves M, Hsu S, et al. Safety and radiation dosimetry profiles of intrathecal I-131 sodium iodide (NaI) in patients with leptomeningeal metastasis (LM) [abstract 3107]. ASCO Annual Meeting Proceedings. J Clin Oncol 2005;23(16s).

73. Kramer K, Humm JL, Souweidane MM, et al. Phase I study of targeted radioimmunotherapy for leptomeningeal cancers using intra-Ommaya 131-I-3F8. J Clin Oncol 2007;25(34):5465–70.

74. Rubenstein JL, Combs D, Rosenberg J, et al. Rituximab therapy for CNS lymphomas: targeting the leptomeningeal compartment. Blood 2003; 101(2):466–8.

75. Rubenstein JL, Fridlyand J, Abrey L, et al. Phase I study of intraventricular administration of rituximab in patients with recurrent CNS and intraocular lymphoma. J Clin Oncol 2007;25(11):1350–6.

76. Jaime-Perez JC, Rodriguez-Romo LN, Gonzalez-Llano O, et al. Effectiveness of intrathecal rituximab in patients with acute lymphoblastic leukaemia relapsed to the CNS and resistant to conventional therapy. Br J Haematol 2009;144(5):794–5.

77. Stemmler HJ, Schmitt M, Willems A, et al. Ratio of trastuzumab levels in serum and cerebrospinal fluid is altered in HER2-positive breast cancer patients with brain metastases and impairment of blood-brain barrier. Anticancer Drugs 2007;18(1):23–8.

78. Laufman LR, Forsthoefel KF. Use of intrathecal trastuzumab in a patient with carcinomatous meningitis. Clin Breast Cancer 2001;2(3):235.

79. Platini C, Long J, Walter S. Meningeal carcinomatosis from breast cancer treated with intrathecal trastuzumab. Lancet Oncol 2006;7(9):778–80.

80. Stemmler HJ, Schmitt M, Harbeck N, et al. Application of intrathecal trastuzumab (Herceptin™) for treatment of meningeal carcinomatosis in HER2-overexpressing metastatic breast cancer. Oncol Rep 2006;15(5):1373–7.

81. Allison DL, Glantz M, Werner TL, et al. Intra-CSF trastuzumab in patients with neoplastic meningitis from breast cancer or primary brain tumors [abstract 2066]. ASCO Annual Meeting Proceedings. J Clin Oncol 2009;27(15s).

82. Hill FG, Richards S, Gibson B, et al. Successful treatment without cranial radiotherapy of children receiving intensified chemotherapy for acute lymphoblastic leukaemia: results of the risk-stratified randomized central nervous system treatment trial MRC UKALL XI (ISRC TN 16757172). Br J Haematol 2004;124(1):33–46.

83. Hill QA, Owen RG. CNS prophylaxis in lymphoma: who to target and what therapy to use. Blood Rev 2006;20(6):319–32.

84. Heideman RL, Cole DE, Balis F, et al. Phase I and pharmacokinetic evaluation of thiotepa in the cerebrospinal fluid and plasma of pediatric patients: evidence for dose-dependent plasma clearance of thiotepa. Cancer Res 1989;49(3):736–41.

85. Vassal G, Gouyette A, Hartmann O, et al. Pharmacokinetics of high-dose busulfan in children. Cancer Chemother Pharmacol 1989;24(6):386–90.

86. Ostermann S, Csajka C, Buclin T, et al. Plasma and cerebrospinal fluid population pharmacokinetics of temozolomide in malignant glioma patients. Clin Cancer Res 2004;10(11):3728–36.

87. Grygiel JJ, Balis FM, Collins JM, et al. Pharmacokinetics of tiazofurin in the plasma and cerebrospinal fluid of rhesus monkeys. Cancer Res 1985;45(5):2037–9.

88. Zimm S, Ettinger LJ, Holcenberg JS, et al. Phase I and clinical pharmacological study of mercaptopurine administered as a prolonged intravenous infusion. Cancer Res 1985;45(4):1869–73.

89. Kerr IG, Zimm S, Collins JM, et al. Effect of intravenous dose and schedule on cerebrospinal fluid pharmacokinetics of 5-fluorouracil in the monkey. Cancer Res 1984;44(11):4929–32.

90. Heideman RL, Balis FM, McCully C, et al. Preclinical pharmacology of arabinosyl-5-azacytidine in nonhuman primates. Cancer Res 1988;48(15):4294–8.

91. Balis FM, Poplack DG. Central nervous system pharmacology of antileukemic drugs. Am J Pediatr Hematol Oncol 1989;11(1):74–86.

92. Slevin ML, Piall EM, Aherne GW, et al. Effect of dose and schedule on pharmacokinetics of high-dose cytosine arabinoside in plasma and cerebrospinal fluid. J Clin Oncol 1983;1(9):546–51.

93. Baker SD, Heideman RL, Crom WR, et al. Cerebrospinal fluid pharmacokinetics and penetration of continuous infusion topotecan in children with central nervous system tumors. Cancer Chemother Pharmacol 1996;37(3):195–202.

94. Beckloff GL, Lerner HJ, Frost D, et al. Hydroxyurea (NSC-32065) in biologic fluids: dose-concentration relationship. Cancer Chemother Rep 1965;48:57–8.

95. Yule SM, Price L, Pearson AD, et al. Cyclophosphamide and ifosfamide metabolites in the cerebrospinal fluid of children. Clin Cancer Res 1997;3(11):1985–92.

96. Blaney SM, Balis FM, Berg S, et al. Intrathecal mafosfamide: a preclinical pharmacology and phase I trial. J Clin Oncol 2005;23(7):1555–63.

97. Blaney SM, Boyett J, Friedman H, et al. Phase I clinical trial of mafosfamide in infants and children aged 3 years or younger with newly diagnosed embryonal tumors: a Pediatric Brain Tumor Consortium study (PBTC-001). J Clin Oncol 2005;23(3):525–31.

98. Gururangan S, Petros WP, Poussaint TY, et al. Phase I trial of intrathecal spartaject busulfan in children with neoplastic meningitis: a Pediatric Brain Tumor Consortium Study (PBTC-004). Clin Cancer Res 2006;12(5):1540–6.

99. Quinn JA, Glantz M, Petros W, et al. Intrathecal spartaject busulfan phase I trial for patients with neoplastic meningitis. Neuro Oncol 2001;3(4):364.

100. Nakagawa H, Miyahara E, Suzuki T, et al. Continuous intrathecal administration of 5-fluoro-2′-deoxyuridine for the treatment of neoplastic meningitis. Neurosurgery 2005;57(2):266–80.

Neurocognitive and Quality of Life Measures in Patients with Metastatic Brain Disease

Mariana E. Witgert, PhD*, Christina A. Meyers, PhD, ABPP

KEYWORDS

• Brain metastasis • Cognition • Quality of life

Brain metastases are the most common intracranial tumors, occurring in 20% to 40% of all patients with cancer.[1] The prognosis for patients with brain metastases is poor, with a median survival of just 1 month if left untreated[2] and 2 to 7 months if treated.[3] The World Health Organization has long defined health as not only the absence of disease but also "complete physical, mental, and social well being."[4] However, perhaps because of the limited survival time associated with brain metastases, much research to date has ignored factors such as cognitive functioning and quality of life (QOL). Instead, most clinical trials have focused on survival, radiological response, and time to disease recurrence. Despite, or even arguably because of, the poor prognosis for these patients, neurocognitive function and QOL are important considerations in assessing the risks and benefits of potential treatments, informing treatment decisions, and maintaining patient functioning for as long as possible. The need to consider these factors is illustrated by Tannock's statement, "When cure is elusive, it is time to start treating the patient and not the tumor."[5] Recently, there has been an increased awareness on both the importance and the feasibility of including cognitive and QOL indices as additional clinical end points.[6] Moving beyond length of survival or presence or absence of disease, measures assessing neurocognitive functioning and QOL are increasingly incorporated into research trials and clinical care.

ASSESSMENT OF NEUROCOGNITIVE IMPAIRMENT IN PATIENTS WITH BRAIN METASTASES

To determine the potential effect of cancer treatment on a patient's pattern of cognitive strengths and weaknesses, objective assessment of cognitive functioning via comprehensive neuropsychological assessment is necessary. In determining whether a specific anticancer therapy is associated with risks or benefits to neurocognitive functioning, it is critical to have information regarding the presence and pattern of neurocognitive impairments before treatment. In patients with brain metastases, neurocognitive impairment is often evident before the initiation of therapies specifically aimed at treating the metastases; the nature and severity of such impairment may be influenced by lesion location, lesion momentum, and the untoward effect of tumor and edema on frontal-subcortical networks. In addition, patients may have already experienced alterations in neurocognitive functioning secondary to the untoward effect of their primary cancer and systemic therapies. In a small pilot study investigating neurocognitive impairment in patients with brain metastases, baseline impairment was observed on at least

The authors have nothing to disclose.

Section of Neuropsychology, Department of Neuro-Oncology, Unit 431, University of Texas MD Anderson Cancer Center, PO Box 301402, Houston, TX 77230-1402, USA

* Corresponding author.

E-mail address: mwitgert@mdanderson.org

Neurosurg Clin N Am 22 (2011) 79–85

doi:10.1016/j.nec.2010.08.010

1042-3680/11/$ — see front matter © 2011 Elsevier Inc. All rights reserved.

one test in 67% of the study population, with most impairment frequently observed on measures assessing executive functioning, motor dexterity, and learning and memory.[7] In the absence of this baseline information, patients might have easily been misclassified as cognitively impaired or not impaired after treatment, and determination of change secondary to subsequent treatment would not have been feasible.

In addition to alterations in neurocognitive functioning secondary to tumors, specific treatments aimed at controlling brain metastases may lead to additional neurocognitive changes. For many years, whole brain radiotherapy (WBRT) was the standard treatment of brain metastases. Recent advances in treatment have revealed a survival benefit of surgery or stereotactic radiosurgery (SRS) plus WBRT over WBRT alone for patients with a single brain metastasis.[8,9] Questions have since been raised regarding the potentially differential effect of these treatments on neurocognitive functioning, with concern that WBRT is potentially more neurotoxic and may even lead to radiation-induced dementia.[10] One study found that WBRT may actually have a beneficial effect on specific aspects of neurocognitive functioning through a reduction in intracranial tumor burden; in this study, patients with a good radiologic response to WBRT showed improvement in performance on tests assessing executive functioning and fine motor dexterity. However, performance on memory testing was not significantly improved, even for those patients with a good radiographic response, and the investigators speculated that hippocampally mediated functions such as memory may be particularly vulnerable to WBRT.[11] Evidence of differential neurotoxicity on memory systems was further demonstrated in a randomized controlled trial, which found that patients receiving SRS plus WBRT were significantly more likely to evidence a decline in learning and memory at 4 months after treatment than patients receiving SRS alone. As a result of the information provided by the inclusion of neurocognitive tests as an outcome measure, the investigators recommended that the initial treatment of brain metastases be limited to the use of SRS alone, with close clinical monitoring for recurrent brain metastases in an effort to preserve neurocognitive functioning for as long as possible.[12]

In addition to providing information regarding potential neurotoxicities associated with treatment, neurocognitive evaluation offers a means to evaluate the effect of therapies that may be beneficial to neurocognitive function in that they may delay expected disease progression. For example, time to neurocognitive progression was prolonged in patients with brain metastases who were treated with WBRT plus motexafin gadolinium, as opposed to WBRT alone.[13]

Feasibility of Neurocognitive Assessment

The complexities involved in assessing the neurocognitive functioning of patients with cancer have been described by Wefel and colleagues,[14] who note that although the administration of objective measures is relatively simple, the selection and interpretation of appropriate measures requires greater knowledge and skill. Test selection varies as a function of the question being asked; in the case of patients with cancer, it is important to select measures that are sensitive to subtle changes in functioning in the cognitive domains that are most likely to be affected by cancer and its treatment. Measures should be reliable and valid, as well as robust to practice effects, because patients are often tested multiple times within a short time span. Alternative test forms, when available, should be used. In the past, such an approach was not consistently used. Rather, the assessment of cognitive functioning in clinical and research settings was all too often limited to brief screening measures, such as the Mini-Mental State Examination (MMSE). The poor sensitivity of this tool for patients with cancer has been documented[15]; comprehensive neuropsychological assessment revealed cognitive impairment in 52 of 67 consecutive patients with brain tumor, whereas MMSE scores were considered abnormal in only 26 of the 52 patients with impairment. Similarly, whereas MMSE scores remained essentially unchanged in a study evaluating the potential neurotoxicity of a mitotic inhibitor, memory function, as measured by a brief word list learning test, declined significantly after each infusion of the agent.[16] In the past, concerns had been raised regarding the feasibility of including a battery of more sensitive neurocognitive measures in the evaluation of patients with brain metastases; these included test administration time, training of staff, and perceived burden on the patient. However, these concerns have been conclusively dismissed; it has been shown that patients are accepting of and compliant with neuropsychological assessment, and inclusion of such assessments has been proven to be feasible in clinical practice and in several research trials,[17,18] with compliance rates for administration and completion actually exceeding those of previous trials using the MMSE alone.[18] Even a brief battery of neurocognitive tests, requiring only approximately 30 minutes to administer, has been shown to be effective in identifying the risk and benefits associated with various anticancer therapies.[17,19] Such a battery has been used in several studies investigating neurocognitive functioning in patients with brain metastases[7,12,17] and includes sensitive tests of learning and memory, attention, processing speed, verbal fluency, executive functioning, and motor dexterity. **Table 1** lists the neurocognitive tests that meet the criteria described earlier and that have been commonly used in trials; these measures involve standardized assessment by either a neuropsychologist or a trained staff member and have published normative data that take into account age, education, and gender, as appropriate.

The utility of neurocognitive assessment in patients with cancer is underscored by evidence demonstrating that cognitive impairment, when documented via formal neuropsychological testing, predicts survival better than clinical prognostic factors alone in patients with primary brain tumors,[25] leptomeningeal disease,[26] and parenchymal brain metastases.[13] Furthermore, Meyers and Hess[6] demonstrated that cognitive performance was a more sensitive predictor of time to tumor progression than magnetic resonance imaging because cognitive decline occurred an average of 6 weeks before radiographic failure in 80 patients with glioblastoma multiforme and anaplastic astrocytoma.

In addition to the above-mentioned considerations, a thorough neurocognitive assessment includes an assessment of the indirect effects of cancer on physical and emotional well-being and the consequent effect of such symptoms on cognitive functioning. Patients with brain metastases may experience neurologic symptoms, sleep disturbance, mood disturbance, pain, and fatigue. Fatigue is generally unrelieved by rest and can have pervasive effects on motivation and action. Mental and physical fatigue can affect cognitive functioning, as can numerous medications and associated medical complications. The reverse can also occur, with cognitive impairment leading to affective distress and fatigue (see Valentine and Meyers[27] for a more thorough review). In cancer populations, self-reporting of cognitive impairment has been shown to correlate more closely with fatigue and mood disturbance than with objective evidence of cognitive dysfunction, as assessed by standardized neuropsychological tests.[28–31] Thus, a thorough neuropsychological assessment is needed to elucidate whether subjectively perceived difficulties are secondary to cancer-related cognitive dysfunction and/or affective distress and fatigue.

ASSESSMENT OF QOL IN PATIENTS WITH BRAIN METASTASES

Although there is no universally accepted definition of QOL, it is generally agreed that QOL is a multidimensional construct encompassing patient perception of overall well-being. It is necessary to differentiate QOL from symptom assessment, because the perceived effect of a given symptom may vary significantly between individuals and over time.[32] QOL data may serve to increase the awareness on variables that affect patient well-being, inform treatment decisions, and identify targets for intervention.[33]

Similar to the assessment of neurocognitive functioning, assessment of patients' QOL has been evolving over time. Historically, most studies used a rating of functional status determined by health care providers, such as the Karnofsky Performance Scale (KPS),[34] as a proxy for QOL. Despite the limited reliability of this scale, which in one study was found to have interphysician agreement of only 29%,[35] it remains the most common outcome measure used in the neuro-oncology literature. In fact, in a review of trials investigating the effect of WBRT on patients with brain metastases, 33 of the 55 trials used the KPS.[36] The KPS, although valuable as a gross estimate of functional status, measures only one facet of the broader concept of QOL. A thorough assessment extending beyond functional status alone can enrich physicians' understanding of

Table 1
Neurocognitive tests commonly used in patients with brain metastases

Cognitive Domain	Test
Learning/Memory	Hopkins Verbal Learning Test—Revised[20]
Attention	WAIS-III Digit Span[21]
Information Processing Speed	Trail Making Test Part A[22] WAIS-III Digit Symbol[21]
Verbal Fluency	Controlled Oral Word Association[23]
Executive Functioning	Trail Making Test Part B[22]
Fine Motor Dexterity	Grooved Pegboard[24]

Abbreviation: WAIS, Wechsler Adult Intelligence Scale.

patient QOL by increasing awareness of other key factors contributing to this outcome.

It must be acknowledged that there are challenges associated with assessing patients' QOL. One of the greatest challenges is the possibility that functional impairment may affect an individual's ability to complete self-report measures; the developers of the Functional Assessment of Cancer Therapy-Brain (FACT-BR), for example, noted that often only higher-functioning patients (KPS>60) are able to complete the questionnaire.[37] Neurocognitive dysfunction may interfere with the patients' ability to accurately complete self-report measures, especially as the disease progresses and cognitive impairment becomes increasingly problematic.[6] Because of these challenges, the use of proxy ratings is inherently appealing, particularly because some patients with brain metastases may be unable to complete self-report measures. Some studies have attempted to garner greater outcome data by including standard measures completed by health care providers or caregiver ratings. However, these approaches are problematic because evidence suggests that patient QOL as rated by physicians and caregivers may be inaccurate. In one study investigating QOL ratings in patients with skull base tumors, surgeons overrated patients' QOL in most cases and there was no significant correlation between patient and surgeon ratings at the individual level.[38] Some data examining patient-caregiver agreement in QOL ratings were initially more encouraging. For example, one study found that substantial discrepancies occurred in only a small minority (5%–10%) of patient-caregiver pairs using the European Organization for Research into the Treatment of Cancer Core Quality of Life Questionnaire (EORTC QLQ-C30).[39] However, the investigators acknowledged that the rating agreement decreased as the patients' level of physical and cognitive impairment increased, leaving questions regarding the reliability of proxy ratings for those who may need them most.[40] In a study examining patient-caregiver agreement for patients with brain metastases, 60 patient-caregiver pairs completed the FACT-BR at baseline (before undergoing WBRT). Concordance between patient and proxy ratings was poor across all scales and could not be determined at follow-up secondary to high rates of attrition.[41] These findings suggest that the use of proxy ratings to assess patient QOL should generally be avoided.

Given that proxy ratings are unlikely to yield consistently accurate information regarding a patient's perceived well-being, the use of patient-reported outcomes has become increasingly recognized as the standard in QOL assessment. An ideal QOL measure can be completed by individuals who may be ill or have mild neurocognitive impairment, demonstrates reliability and validity, and taps patient perception of all relevant domains, including functional status, social well-being, cognitive symptoms, physical functioning, and emotional health. Although no perfect or universally applicable measure exists, numerous instruments have been developed in an effort to meet the need for QOL data in patients with cancer and several have been applied in patients with brain metastases.

One of the most commonly used QOL instruments is the FACT,[42] a self-report instrument that provides information regarding patient's perceptions of their physical, social, emotional, and functional well-being. An additional subscale addressing issues relevant to patients with brain tumors was also developed (FACT-BR)[37]; both the general scale and the brain subscale have been demonstrated to have good validity and reliability. In one study investigating the effect of WBRT on patient-rated QOL, a statistically nonsignificant mean deterioration in FACT-BR ratings was observed from baseline to 1 month.[43] Similarly, a more recent study showed a trend toward worsening FACT-BR ratings at 2 months post-WBRT; some patients were unable to complete the questionnaire at the later time point secondary to significant health declines or death.[41]

Other QOL measures have also indicated a decline in QOL after treatment of brain metastases. A recent pilot study used the EORTC QLQ-C30,[39] a validated measure including domains assessing physical, cognitive, emotional, and social functioning, as well as global QOL, symptoms, and financial consequences. A shortened version of the questionnaire, the QLQ-C15-PAL, was also used. Combined data from these measures revealed relatively stable ratings of global QOL but declines in physical functioning, energy level, and appetite.[44]

Although the above-mentioned studies suggest a trend toward declining QOL in association with WBRT for brain metastases, other studies yield a different finding. For example, a small study including 19 patients with brain metastases who had received surgery or radiosurgery for a solitary brain metastasis and who were randomized to receive WBRT versus observation found no difference in change from baseline in patient QOL ratings on the EORTC QLQ-C30. It is noted, however, that the analyses in this study included only the 2 global questions regarding overall health and QOL.[45] Another study found significant improvement across all parameters measured by the EORTC QLC-C30, including global QOL, perceived physical,role, emotional, cognitive, and social functioning as well as improvement in many symptoms.[46]

ASSOCIATION BETWEEN NEUROCOGNITIVE FUNCTIONING AND QOL

Changes in QOL do not parallel changes in neurocognitive functioning and, therefore, cannot be used as a proxy for thorough assessment of cognitive abilities. However, a link between neurocognitive functioning and self-reported QOL has been demonstrated in patients with brain metastases. In one study, a strong correlation was observed between memory and executive functioning, as measured by objective neuropsychological tests, and patient-reported QOL, as measured by ratings on the FACT-BR. This correlation was present at baseline and remained significant after patients received WBRT. Declines in neurocognitive functioning were evident before declines in patient ratings of QOL, with deterioration of performance on a memory test proving to be the strongest predictor of subsequent declines in patient-reported QOL.[47]

INTERVENTIONS FOR NEUROCOGNITIVE AND QOL CONCERNS

In addition to providing information regarding potential neurotoxicities associated with brain metastases and antineoplastic therapies, as well as the effect of those toxicities on patient well-being, information gained through assessment of neurocognitive functioning and QOL offers an opportunity to identify potential points of intervention. Interventions designed to minimize the adverse cognitive and emotional consequences of the disease and treatment offer a significant opportunity to improve the QOL of patients, regardless of the stage of their illness. A multidisciplinary approach incorporating pharmacologic, cognitive, behavioral, and rehabilitative therapies has the potential to maximize everyday functioning, coping, and adjustment, with the ultimate goal of maintaining the highest level of functioning for the longest possible time.

Pharmacologic intervention includes the use of antidepressants to address affective distress. Stimulant medications have also been shown to be effective in addressing fatigue and cognitive dysfunction in patients with cancer and were helpful in elevating mood.[48] Even a conservative dose of 10 mg twice a day significantly improved cognitive function as assessed by objective tests, and doses in excess of 60 mg twice a day were well

tolerated. Subjective improvements included improved gait, increased stamina and motivation to perform activities, and improved bladder control. There were no significant side effects, and many patients taking steroids were able to decrease their dose.

Psychosocial interventions have also been shown to have a positive effect on QOL in adult patients with cancer; evidence suggests that many different forms of intervention are beneficial.[49] Some of the more common approaches are individual psychotherapy or counseling, support groups (professionally facilitated or peer led), and psychoeducational activities to explain potential neurobehavioral symptoms.

Compensatory strategies, traditionally studied in the context of rehabilitation with stroke and traumatic brain injury, have also been used; generally, such interventions involve training in the use of external compensatory tools, stress management, energy conservation, and psychoeducation, as well as accommodations in the patient's home and hospital environment to increase structure and decrease demands for planning and decision making. Even patients in terminal care can benefit from methods to enhance their orientation and social interactions.

Continued research into the mechanisms of treatment-related cognitive dysfunction may afford opportunities for the development of neuroprotective therapies, effective adjuvant supportive pharmacotherapies, and/or modification of primary treatments. In addition, advances in neuropsychological interventions will help minimize the effect of cancer and cancer therapy on neurocognitive function, QOL, and functional abilities. As primary therapy becomes more effective and more patients experience long-term remissions, assessment of neurobehavioral function and QOL and establishment of targeted and effective treatment strategies will gain even greater importance.

SUMMARY

The assessment of neurocognitive function and QOL in patients with brain metastases has become increasingly recognized as an important addition to traditional outcome measures such as length of survival and time to disease progression. Changes in cognitive functioning and QOL may arise as a consequence of tumor growth or as an adverse side effect of necessary antineoplastic treatments. Merely assessing functional status is not sufficient to assay these outcomes, as this is only a facet of a larger complex domain. Neurocognitive assessment should include baseline evaluations to determine whether observed patterns of performance represent a change from premorbid levels; evaluations should include sensitive measures assessing the various cognitive domains known to be affected by cancer and cancer treatment, including learning and memory, processing speed, executive functioning, and fine motor control. Although objective assessment of neurocognitive function using standardized neuropsychological tests is well established, QOL represents a more subjective concept for which no gold standard assessment tool has been identified. Data suggest that QOL measures should focus on patient self-report because health care providers and caregivers may be unable to serve as accurate proxies for this subjective experience of well-being. Patient-reported outcomes of QOL should have established reliability and validity and should tap the various aspects of QOL, including physical, emotional, and social functioning, as well as functional status and symptoms specific to the disease and treatment. A thorough evaluation of these factors is useful for assessing baseline (ie, pretreatment) cognitive functioning and QOL, monitoring the effects of cancer and cancer treatment on these outcomes, allowing comparison of available treatments and informing future treatment decisions, and facilitating development and planning of behavioral and pharmacologic interventions to minimize the effect of symptoms on functional well-being.

REFERENCES

1. Soffietti R, Ruda R, Mutani R. Management of brain metastases. J Neurol 2002;249:1357–69.
2. Tosoni A, Ermani M, Brandes AA. The pathogenesis and treatment of brain metastases: a comprehensive review. Crit Rev Oncol Hematol 2004;52:199–215.
3. Gaspar L, Scott C, Rotman M, et al. Recursive partitioning analysis (RPA) of prognostic factors in three radiation therapy oncology group (RTOG) brain metastases trials. Int J Radiat Oncol Biol Phys 1997;37:745–75.
4. Preamble to the Constitution of the World Health Organization as adopted by the International Health Conference, New York, 19-22 June, 1946; signed on 22 July 1946 by the representatives of 61 States (Official Records of the World Health Organization, no. 2, p. 100) and entered into force on 7 April 1948. Available at: http://www.who.int/about/definition/en/print.html/. Accessed May 3, 2010.
5. Tannock IF. Treating the patient, not just the cancer. N Engl J Med 1987;317:1534–5.
6. Meyers CA, Hess KR. Multifaceted end points in brain tumor clinical trials: cognitive deterioration precedes MRI progression. Neuro Oncol 2003;5: 89–95.
7. Chang EL, Wefel JS, Maor MH, et al. A pilot study of neurocognitive function in patients with one to three new brain metastases initially treated with stereotactic radiosurgery alone. Neurosurgery 2007;60:277–84.
8. Andrews DW, Scott CB, Sperduto PW, et al. Whole brain radiation therapy with or without stereotactic radiosurgery boost for patients with one to three brain metastases: phase III results of the RTOG 9508 randomised trial. Lancet 2004;363:1665–72.
9. Patchell R, Tibbs P, Walsh J, et al. A randomized trial of surgery in the treatment of single metastases to the brain. N Engl J Med 1990;322:494–500.
10. DeAngelis LM, Delattre J, Posner JB. Radiation-induced dementia in patients cured of brain metastases. Neurology 1989;39:789–96.
11. Li J, Bentzen SM, Renschler M, et al. Regression after whole-brain radiation therapy for brain metastases correlates with survival and improved neurocognitive function. J Clin Oncol 2007;25:1260–6.
12. Chang EL, Wefel JS, Hess KR, et al. Neurocognition in patients with brain metastases treated with radiosurgery or radiosurgery plus whole-brain irradiation: a randomized controlled trial. Lancet Oncol 2009;10: 1037–44.
13. Meyers CA, Smith JA, Bezjak A, et al. Neurocognitive function and progression in patients with brain metastases treated with whole-brain radiation and motexafin gadolinium: results of a randomized phase III trial. J Clin Oncol 2004;22:157–65.
14. Wefel JS, Kayl AE, Meyers CA. Neuropsychological dysfunction associated with cancer and cancer therapies: a conceptual review of an emerging target. Br J Cancer 2004;90:1691–6.
15. Meyers CA, Wefel JS. The use of the mini-mental state examination to assess cognitive functioning in cancer trials: no ifs, ands, buts, or sensitivity. J Clin Oncol 2003;21:3557–8.
16. Meyers CA, Kudelka AP, Conrad CA, et al. Neurotoxicity of CI-980, a novel mitotic inhibitor. Clin Cancer Res 1997;3:419–22.
17. Herman MA, Tremont-Lukats I, Meyers CA, et al. Neurocognitive and functional assessment of patients with brain metastasis: a pilot study. Am J Clin Oncol 2003;26:273–9.
18. Regine WF, Schmitt FA, Scott CB, et al. Feasibility of neurocognitive outcome evaluations in patients with brain metastases in a multi-institutional cooperative group setting: results of radiation therapy oncology group trial BR-0018. Int J Radiat Oncol Biol Phys 2004;58:1346–52.
19. Meyers CA, Brown PD. Role and relevance of neurocognitive assessment in clinical trials of patients with CNS tumors. J Clin Oncol 2006;8:1305–9.
20. Benedict RH, Schretlen D, Groniger L, et al. Hopkins Verbal Learning Test — revised: normative data and analysis of inter-form and test-retest reliability. Clin Neuropsychol 1998;12:43–55.

21. Wechsler D. WAIS-III administration and scoring manual. San Antonio (TX): The Psychological Corporation; 1997.

22. Army Individual Test Battery. Manual of directions and scoring. Washington, DC: War Department, Adjutant General's Office; 1944.

23. Benton AL, Hamscher KD. Multilingual aphasia examination. Iowa City (IA): AJA Associates; 1989.

24. Reitan RM, Davison LA. Clinical neuropsychology: current status and applications. Washington, DC: VH Winston & Sons; 1974.

25. Meyers CA, Hess KR, Yung WK, et al. Cognitive function as a predictor of survival in patients with recurrent malignant glioma. J Clin Oncol 2000;18:646–50.

26. Sherman AM, Jaeckle K, Meyers CA. Pre-treatment cognitive performance predicts survival in patients with leptomeningeal disease. Cancer 2002;95:1311–66.

27. Valentine AD, Meyers CA. Cognitive and mood disturbance as causes and symptoms of fatigue in cancer patients. Cancer 2001;92:1694–8.

28. Castellon SA, Ganz PA, Bower JE, et al. Neurocognitive performance in breast cancer survivors exposed to adjuvant chemotherapy and tamoxifen. J Clin Exp Neuropsychol 2004;26:955–69.

29. Jenkins V, Shilling V, Deutsch G, et al. A 3-year prospective study of the effects of adjuvant treatments on cognition in women with early stage breast cancer. Br J Cancer 2006;94:828–34.

30. Schagen SB, Muller MJ, Boogerd W, et al. Cognitive dysfunction and chemotherapy: neuropsychological findings in perspective. Clin Breast Cancer 2002;3-(Suppl. 3):S100–8.

31. Houston WS, Bondi MW. Potentially reversible cognitive symptoms in older adults. In: Attik DK, Welsh-Bohmer KA, editors. Geriatric neuropsychology assessment and intervention. New York: Guilford Press; 2006. p. 103–31.

32. Murphy BA, Ridner S, Wells N, et al. Quality of life research in head and neck cancer: a review of the current state of the science. Crit Rev Oncol Hematol 2007;62:251–67.

33. Gil Z, Abergel A, Spektor S, et al. Patient, caregiver, and surgeon perceptions of quality of life following anterior skull base surgery. Arch Otolaryngol Head Neck Surg 2004;130:1276–81.

34. Karnofsky DA, Burchenal JH. The clinical evaluation of chemotherapeutic agents in cancer. In: McLeod CM, editor. Evaluation of chemotherapeutic agents. New York: Columbia University Press; 1949. p. 191–205.

35. Hutchison TA, Boyd NF, Feinstein AR. Scientific problems in clinical scales, as demonstrated in the Karnofsky Index of Performance Status. J Chronic Dis 1979;32:661–6.

36. Wong J, Hird A, Kirou-Mauro A, et al. Quality of life in brain metastases radiation trials: a literature review. Curr Oncol 2008;15:25–45.

37. Weitzner MA, Meyers CA, Gelke CK, et al. The Functional Assessment of Cancer Therapy (FACT) scale. Development of a brain subscale and revalidation of the general version (FACT-G) in patients with primary brain tumors. Cancer 1995;75:1151–61.

38. Steinvorth S, Welzel G, Fuss M, et al. Neuropsychological outcome after fractionated stereotactic radiotherapy (FSRT) for base of skull meningiomas: a prospective 1-year follow-up. Radiother Oncol 2003;69:177–82.

39. Aaronson NK, Ahmedzai S, Bergman B, et al. The European Organization for Research and Treatment of Cancer QLQ-C30: a quality of life instrument for use in international clinical trials in oncology. J Natl Cancer Inst 1993;85:365–76.

40. Sneeuw KC, Aaronson NK, Osoba D, et al. The use of significant others as proxy raters of the quality of life of patients with brain cancer. Med Care 1997;35:490–506.

41. Doyle M, Bradley NM, Li K, et al. Quality of life in patients with brain metastases treated with a palliative course of whole-brain radiotherapy. J Palliat Med 2007;10:367–74.

42. Cella DF, Tulsky DS, Gray G, et al. The functional assessment of cancer therapy scale: development and validation of the general measure. J Clin Oncol 1993;11:570–9.

43. Bezjak A, Adam J, Barton R, et al. Symptom response after palliative radiotherapy for patients with brain metastases. Eur J Cancer 2002;38:487–96.

44. Steinmann D, Schäfer C, van Oorschot B, et al. Effects of radiotherapy for brain metastases on quality of life (QoL). Strahlenther Onkol 2009;185:190–7.

45. Roos DE, Wirth A, Burmeister BH, et al. Whole brain irradiation following surgery or radiosurgery for solitary brain metastases: mature results of a prematurely closed randomized Trans-Tasman Radiation Oncology Group Trial (TROG 98.05). Radiother Oncol 2006;80:318–22.

46. Yaneva M, Semerdjieva M. Assessment of the effect of palliative radiotherapy for cancer patients with intracranial metastases using EORTC-QOL-C30 questionnaire. Folia Med 2006;48:23–9.

47. Li J, Bentzen SM, Li J, et al. Relationship between neurocognitive function and quality of life after whole-brain radiotherapy in patients with brain metastasis. Int J Radiat Oncol Biol Phys 2008;71:64–70.

48. Meyers CA, Weitzner MA, Valentine AD, et al. Methylphenidate improves cognition, mood, and function of brain tumor patients. J Clin Oncol 1998;16:2522–7.

49. Rehse B, Pukrop R. Effects of psychosocial interventions on quality of life in adult cancer patients: meta analysis of 37 published controlled outcome studies. Patient Educ Couns 2003;50:179–86.

Investigational Therapies for Brain Metastases

Muhammad M. Abd-El-Barr, MD, PhD[a],
Maryam Rahman, MD, MS[a], Ganesh Rao, MD[b],*

KEYWORDS

• Brain metastases • Therapy • Surgery • Chemotherapy

Approximately 1 million Americans are diagnosed with cancer every year, and approximately 1 out of every 2 men and 1 out of every 3 women have some type of cancer during their lifetime (www.cancer.org). The true incidence of brain metastasis is difficult to accurately ascertain because many patients who are neurologically asymptomatic do not undergo routine neuroimaging.[1] A modest estimate of the true incidence of brain metastasis from cancer suggests that one-third of patients with systemic cancer or approximately 200,000 patients every year in the United States have metastasis of the brain.[2] When compared with primary brain tumors, with an incidence estimated to be 20,000 persons[3] in the United States, metastatic brain tumors are much more common. Contrary to the incidence of primary cancers, the incidence of brain metastasis has been increasing. This increase is likely because of the effects of an aging population, improved neuroimaging surveillance, and better control of systemic cancer, allowing time for brain metastasis to occur. Metastatic brain tumors have the capacity to bypass the blood-brain barrier, which provides them a harbor for unmitigated growth; once in the brain, they are generally protected from the cytotoxic effects of chemotherapy. The mechanism of metastatic growth involves genetic transformation of normal or, perhaps, cancer stem cells into a proliferative mass of tumor, which then gains access to the brain through angiogenesis and to the blood stream (**Fig. 1**).

Unlike systemic cancers, for which chemotherapy is the mainstay of treatment, the therapeutic strategies available to treat brain metastasis have traditionally been limited to surgical resection, whole brain radiation therapy (WBRT), or stereotactic radiosurgery (SRS), either individually or in combination.[4–11] Each of these treatments has their advantages and disadvantages. It is important to put the treatment in the context of the prognosis for patients with brain metastases. At the beginning of the twentieth century, diagnosis of a brain metastasis was a sign of terminal cancer and meant a survival limited to weeks. With the advent of WBRT and glucocorticoids for symptomatic improvement, survival was increased dramatically to 4 to 6 months. Later, in the 1990s, the combination of surgical resection and WBRT was shown to be superior to WBRT alone[12] or surgery alone in high-functioning patients.[6] The median survival was increased to 6 months in patients treated with WBRT alone and 10 months to those treated with surgical resection followed by WBRT. Surgery provides local disease control, especially for large-volume metastatic lesions, and can correct the potentially life-threatening consequences of mass effect and herniation. However, surgery does not protect against progression of disease

The authors have nothing to disclose.
[a] Department of Neurosurgery, University of Florida, Box 100265, Gainesville, FL 32610, USA
[b] Department of Neurosurgery, The University of Texas, MD Anderson Cancer Center, 1515 Holcombe Boulevard, Houston, TX 77030, USA
* Corresponding author.
E-mail address: grao@mdanderson.org

Neurosurg Clin N Am 22 (2011) 87–96
doi:10.1016/j.nec.2010.08.008
1042-3680/11/$ – see front matter © 2011 Elsevier Inc. All rights reserved.

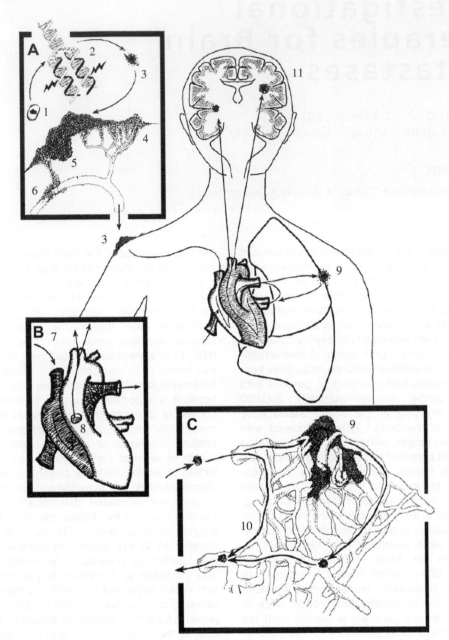

Fig. 1. Pathophysiology of brain metastases. (*A*) A normal cell (**1**) undergoes multiple genetic mutations or epigenetic changes (**2**) to become a cancer (a melanoma as shown here) (**3**). It then proliferates uncontrollably and develops its own feeding vessels (**4**) (angiogenesis), invades the normal tissue stroma (**5**), and enters blood vessels or lymph channels (**6**). (*B*) The tumor gains access to the right side of the heart via the venous circulation (**7**). The cancer cells may be shunted to the left side of the heart via a patent foramen ovale or septal defect (**8**), or (*C*) more commonly, the cancer cells leave the heart via the pulmonary artery to reach the lung capillary bed (**9**), where they may either form a metastasis (**9**) or pass through the capillary bed to reach the left atrium (**10**), from where the tumor cells enter the arterial circulation and seed the brain usually at the gray matter/white matter junction. If the brain is hospitable, the tumor may leave brain capillaries and become a brain metastasis (**11**). (*From* Gavrilovic IT, Posner JB. Brain metastases: epidemiology and pathophysiology. J Neurooncol 2005;75:5–14; with permission.)

at a local site or recurrence at distant sites.[6] Furthermore, some patients may not be suitable surgical candidates because of their systemic disease and/or comorbidities or the location of the metastatic lesions.

With the advent of the Gamma Knife and modifications to the linear accelerator, SRS was introduced as another therapeutic option for patients with brain metastases. SRS with WBRT was found to be equivalent to surgical resection followed by WBRT for smaller lesions (<3 cm) without major mass effect.[13–15] When WBRT is combined with surgical resection or SRS, it has been shown to help decrease local and distant recurrences.[6] However, WBRT has been shown to cause various neurocognitive side effects[16,17] and is indiscriminate in its neurotoxic effects. Still, with the individualized use of these treatment methods, survival with brain metastases has been extended to more than 1 year, and most patients now succumb to systemic effects of their cancer rather than their brain metastases.[18]

It is in the context of the advantages and disadvantages of current therapies that experimental therapies must be judged. In general, the new or experimental treatments are divided into 5 major categories, as proposed by a recent summary of existing treatment options for patients with metastatic brain disease[19]: (1) radiation sensitizers, (2) local irradiation to a resection or biopsy bed, (3) local chemotherapy to the resection or biopsy bed, (4) new chemotherapeutic agents, and (5) therapies that have shown promise in vitro and/or in animal experiments.

RADIATION SENSITIZERS

Because of the indiscriminate neurotoxic effects of WBRT and the associated cognitive side effects,[17] radiation sensitizers are used to make tumor cells more susceptible to radiation while minimizing the exposure of surrounding normal tissue to radiation. Several of these sensitizers have been studied, albeit with mixed results.

Lonidamine, an indazole carboxylic acid derivative, showed promise in in vitro experiments and animals studies as a potent sensitizer of tumor cells to radiation but failed to show any difference in response rate or survival when compared with standard WBRT doses.[20]

Thalidomide, although a potent teratogen, has recently been approved as part of a treatment paradigm for newly diagnosed multiple myeloma. However, it failed to show survival benefit when combined with conventional WBRT as compared with WBRT alone,[21] although these patients had multiple, large, or midbrain metastases.

The 2 most recent sensitizers motexafin gadolinium (MGd) and efaproxiral (RSR13) similarly showed promise in early studies, but their efficacy in randomized controlled trials has been disappointing. However, there are some positive aspects to the agents worth noting.

MGd is a metalloporphyrin with its exact mechanism of action not entirely understood but is thought to increase intracellular levels of reactive oxygen species and hence induce apoptosis in the cells that have taken up MGd. It has been shown to have selective reuptake in tumor cells,[22,23] is able to cross the blood-brain barrier, and because it contains the ferromagnetic material gadolinium, it can be imaged with magnetic resonance imaging. Early phase 1b/2 studies showed that MGd was well tolerated and had very favorable radiological response exceeding 70%.[24] However, a subsequent randomized controlled study comparing MGd and WBRT to WBRT alone failed to show any difference in median survival.[25] Subset analysis revealed that neurologic progression of disease was delayed in the MGd and WBRT combination versus WBRT alone for those patients with lung cancer, but other cancer types did not demonstrate this effect (**Fig. 2**). A subsequent phase 3 study of patients with non–small cell lung carcinoma (NSCLC) failed to show significant differences in time to neurologic progression between patients treated with MGd and WBRT versus WBRT,[26] although it was shown that in those patients treated with MGd and WBRT promptly, there was a significant delay in neurologic progression. Thus, in select patients, namely those with NSCLC that has metastasized to the brain, there may be benefit to administer MGd with WBRT in a prompt manner.

RSR13 is a synthetic substance that causes a conformational change in hemoglobin, decreasing its oxygen-binding affinity resulting in greater oxygen tension and hence greater radiation sensitization.[27] A phase 2 trial of WBRT plus RSR13 resulted in a median survival time of 6.4 months, which was significantly longer than the survival of 4.1 months with WBRT alone from the Radiation Therapy Oncology Group database.[28] A subsequent phase 3 trial failed to show significant differences in survival between RSR13 and WBRT and WBRT alone, although subset analysis showed that there was a significant survival benefit for women with metastatic breast cancer.[29] However, a confirmatory phase 3 trial of women with metastatic breast cancer failed to show significant differences between those treated with RSR13 and WBRT and WBRT alone. Thus, it would seem that although the premise is promising, the use of RSR13 may not be warranted at present.

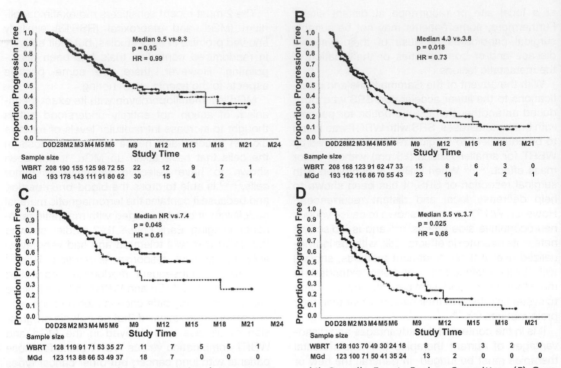

Fig. 2. Time to neurologic progression by treatment arm. (*A*) Overall—Events Review Committee. (*B*) Overall—investigator. (*C*) Lung—Events Review Committee. (*D*) Lung—investigator. Study time is in days (D) or months (M); median is in months. HRs were calculated using Cox proportional hazards model. Abbreviations: HR, hazard ratio; NR, not reached. (*From* Mehta MP, Rodrigus P, Terhaard CH, et al. Survival and neurologic outcomes in a randomized trial of motexafin gadolinium and whole-brain radiation therapy in brain metastases. J Clin Oncol 2003;21:2529–36; with permission.)

LOCAL IRRADIATION

Brachytherapy, which is the placement of radiation sources close to the area being treated, has been used successfully in treating cancers, including prostate,[30] cervical,[31] and breast cancers.[32] The most common brachytherapy source is iodine 125 (^{125}I). The first cohort study comparing ^{125}I seeds and WBRT with ^{125}I seeds alone showed median survival time of 17 and 15 months, respectively, which was not statistically different. Two other case series[33,34] showed efficacy of ^{125}I seeds, but no randomized controlled study has been completed. Other studies have combined surgery and delivery of ^{125}I through the GliaSite Radiation Therapy System (Cytyc Surgical Products II, Mountain View, CA, USA), with mixed results (**Fig. 3**). A phase 2 study showed a median survival of approximately 40 weeks, with local control rate at approximately 80% and distant brain control rate at 50% that are comparable to previous studies of surgery followed by WBRT or SRS. The major concern in this study was the occurrence of

radiation necrosis, which was estimated to be 17%.[35] The investigators suggested that such a therapeutic strategy may be effective in delaying WBRT after resection, thus minimizing toxic effects to the rest of the brain. Other case series[36,37] have shown some positive results, but no randomized controlled study has been completed comparing surgery and local brachytherapy to current standard treatments, including surgery, WBRT, or SRS. Thus, there does seem to be some advantage to local brachytherapy, especially regarding local tumor control and possibly delaying WBRT. However, this advantage may be offset by the increased risk for radiation necrosis.

LOCAL CHEMOTHERAPY

There have been a few studies evaluating the use and efficacy of local chemotherapy to increase local control of brain metastases. A biodegradable biopolymer wafer containing BCNU (carmustine) (marketed as Gliadel in the United States) has shown promising results in the treatment of primary

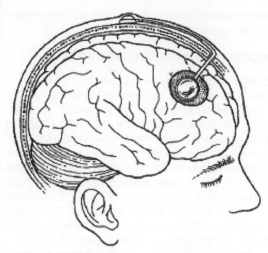

Fig. 3. The GliaSite device. The inflatable balloon catheter is sized to fit the resection cavity. The device was then filled with a radiation source (aqueous ^{125}I radiotherapy solution). After completion of the treatment, the device was removed during a subsequent operation. (*Adapted from* Rogers LR, Rock JP, Sills AK, et al. Results of a phase II trial of the GliaSite radiation therapy system for the treatment of newly diagnosed, resected single brain metastases. J Neurosurg 2006;105(3):377; with permission.)

brain tumors.[38] This wafer has recently been used in the treatment of metastatic brain tumors. In one study, 25 patients with solitary brain metastases were enrolled in a single-arm study of surgical resection, with the use of BCNU wafers and WBRT.[39] Median survival was 33 weeks, and with a median follow-up of 36 weeks, there was no local recurrence of tumor, although distant metastases occurred. Other groups have shown some success with other substances such as 5-fluoro-2'-deoxy-uridine administered with the use of an Ommaya reservoir.[40] To date, no randomized study of local chemotherapy has been published, although the clinical and preclinical data are promising.[39,41]

OTHER LOCAL TREATMENTS

There has been a renewed interest in other local therapies such as photodynamic therapy (PDT) and interstitial radiosurgery. PDT consists of injecting a photosensitizer, a chemical compound that can be excited by application of light of a certain wavelength. Once the photosensitizer is excited, it has the capability of acting as a killer substance.[42] In a prospective trial, 14 patients were treated with PDT and followed up for 70 weeks, with a mean survival of 40 weeks.[43] Again, without a comparable control group, it is difficult to ascertain the true effectiveness of this therapy, although it seems promising. One disadvantage

of this treatment paradigm is that patients must stay out of direct sunlight for an extended period. There have also been numerous reports of local radiosurgery in which a small x-ray generator is placed within difficult-to-reach tumors. These treatments seem to increase local control, but distant metastases are not inhibited.[44,45]

The use of interstitial laser ablation for treatment of brain metastasis was reported as far back as 1992.[46] This technology uses the heat generated by a laser to treat an intracranial brain metastasis. A fiberoptic cable is stereotactically inserted into the tumor to deliver the treatment. Advantages of this treatment include the ability to control the amount of energy delivered and conform the treatment to the specific volume of the lesion.[47] More recently, this treatment has evolved to incorporate the use of nanoparticles to augment the effect of the laser (increasing the amount of heat delivered to the tumor).[48] Nanoshells delivered intravenously diffuse passively into an orthotopic xenograft, and an optical fiber is implanted within the tumor. This process not only augments the amount of thermal energy delivered to the tumor but also minimizes the amount of damage to adjacent normal brain tissues.

SYSTEMIC CHEMOTHERAPY

Apart from local control, as well as control of distant metastases, a third and critical component of treating brain metastasis is securing systemic control of cancer. Although surgical resection of primary site of cancer is a mainstay of treatment, additional treatment often entails the use of chemotherapy. This section does not review chemotherapy aimed at systemic control but concentrates on chemotherapy aimed specifically at brain metastases. The 2 important compounds that have some success in the treatment of brain metastases are temozolomide (TMZ) and fotemustine.

TMZ is an oral alkylating agent that has shown considerable efficacy in treating primary brain tumors, especially glioblastoma multiforme (GBM).[49,50] However, numerous studies have shown that TMZ is promising as a treatment of metastatic brain tumors. Although TMZ is administered orally, it has demonstrated reasonable penetration of the blood-brain barrier.[51] Two randomized phase 2 studies showed benefit in patients who were administered TMZ and WBRT compared with those who received only WBRT, with those who received TMZ demonstrating a greater local response rate and time to progression, although the overall survival times were not significantly different.[52,53] Similar to the fact that the expression of O6-methylguanine-DNA methyltransferase (MGMT) has been shown to correlate with a greater response to TMZ in patients with GBM,[50] a recent study showed that MGMT expression was more likely in metastatic lung cancer than in primary lesions. Positive MGMT expression correlated significantly with longer survival times (**Fig. 4**).[54]

One potentially confounding variable in analyzing the efficacy of any treatment modality in general, and the usefulness of TMZ in treating brain metastases specifically, is that the clinical behavior of metastatic lesions varies by histology. As discussed in a recent review,[19] it seems that brain metastases from lung carcinomas are more amenable to treatment with TMZ. This amenability may be because lung cancer metastases have been shown to express methylated MGMT at a higher rate than other primary cancers.[55]

Fotemustine is an intravenously administered alkylating agent that has shown promise in the treatment of disseminated melanoma.[56] A randomized controlled trial of fotemustine and WBRT versus WBRT alone in patients with metastatic melanoma showed that those patients treated with fotemustine had improved performance status, but no difference in tumor response rate or overall survival was found between the 2 groups.[57]

From this analysis, it is clear that although chemotherapy may play a role in the treatment of brain metastases, it must be done on an

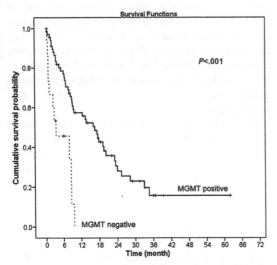

Fig. 4. Kaplan-Meier estimate of overall survival in relation to MGMT expression in brain metastases. (*Adapted from* Wu PF, Kuo KT, Kuo LT, et al. O(6)-Methylguanine-DNA methyltransferase expression and prognostic value in brain metastases of lung cancers. Lung Cancer 2010;68(3):484–90; with permission.)

individualized nature, depending on the primary tumor type and molecular profiling.

MOLECULAR TARGETED THERAPIES

Similar to the study of primary brain tumors, in which genetic and genomic profiling has uncovered molecular targets of interest,[58,59] recent work has revealed important molecular targets in the pathogenesis and therapeutic susceptibility of various brain metastases. One such target is the epidermal growth factor receptor (EGFR) that has been shown to have multiple mutations in brain metastases, especially from NSCLC.[60,61] Gefitinib is an oral tyrosine kinase inhibitor of EGFR and has shown efficacy in the control of brain metastases, particularly if patients harbor an activating mutation or mutations in the tyrosine kinase domain.[61,62] However, no randomized controlled study on the benefit of gefitinib for the treatment of brain metastases has been undertaken. Another feature of brain metastases, which has been exploited for treatment of brain metastases, is increased angiogenesis associated with the tumors.[63] Bevacizumab is a monoclonal antibody that blocks vascular endothelial growth factor A and has been used with good results in GBM as well as retinal proliferation. It has also been shown to have reasonable antitumor effects, especially in NSCLC and breast and colon cancers that have metastasized to the brain.[64,65] There were some concerns that bevacizumab may be associated with increased risk of intracranial hemorrhage,[66] but a large retrospective analysis of several studies suggested that the rate of hemorrhage is more likely because of the metastatic lesion rather than the use of bevacizumab.[67] Other interesting targets for molecular associated therapies include HER2/neu, cyclooxygenase 2, and the alpha-2,6-sialyltransferase ST6GALNAC5 in the pathogenesis of breast cancer metastasizing to the brain.[68,69] In an example of the value of genetic information, a collaborative team was able to identify 51 genes that were overexpressed in patients with breast cancer who were more likely to have brain metastases and 22 more genes correlated with bone metastases.[70] Although some may advocate prophylactic treatment of patients with these genetic profiles, the more elegant and safe method would be to develop inhibitors and/or modulators of the enzymes or proteins encoded by these genes. In the case of NSCLC, gene mining has revealed that the expression of CDH2 (N-cadherin), KIFC1, and FALZ is highly correlated with the development of brain metastases,[71] but again development of inhibitors is still at the experimental and/or developmental stage.

STEM CELL–ASSOCIATED THERAPEUTICS

The utility of stem cell–associated therapies for brain metastases is being investigated. The belief that the adult mammalian brain is unable to generate new brain cells was entrenched in the scientific and medical community for the better part of the last century, despite findings of mitotic cells in the postnatal mammalian brain.[72–74] Reports in the 1950s to 1970s of new neurons being generated in the mature mammalian central nervous system (CNS) were largely ignored.[75–81] One of the confounding problems for the acceptance of continuous neurogenesis in the mammalian CNS was the lack of any evidence of a stem cell population that would sustain new cell genesis throughout the life of the animal. Although several technical advances contributed to studies that overturned the "no new neuron" dogma, the demonstration in 1992 by Reynolds and Weiss[82] that the mature mammalian CNS contained a stem cell population supported the notion that the adult brain had the capacity to generate new cells.

With the widespread recognition of the presence of adult mammalian neural stem/progenitor cells (NSPCs), using these cells therapeutically has become an interesting possibility. Initially used for degenerative diseases of the brain, NSPCs were subsequently used experimentally to deliver therapy to gliomas.[83] NSPCs would localize to intracerebral glioma cells, even when injected into the peripheral circulation.[83] This tumor tropism was then also demonstrated with brain metastasis in vitro.[84] Schmidt and colleagues[84] found that surgical specimen extracts of melanoma and lung and breast cancers induced significant migration of NSPCs, and the magnitude of this finding was dependent on the amount of vascular endothelial growth factor present in these extracts.

Building on these results, Aboody and colleagues[85] described treating melanoma brain tumors with engineered NSPCs in a mouse model. Intracranial melanoma tumors were established in mice by injecting murine melanoma cells into the internal carotid artery. Subsequently, the mice received an internal carotid artery injection of cytosine deaminase (CD)-expressing NSPCs (CD-NSPCs) and systemic 5-fluorocytosine (5-FC). The NSPCs localized to areas of tumor and 5-FC was successfully converted to 5-fluorouracil by the CD expressed on these cells. This process was demonstrated by a significant reduction in tumor size.[85]

Similarly, Joo and colleagues[86] described successful treatment of breast cancer in a mouse model using CD-NSPCs. After establishment of the tumor, the mice received an intracranial injection of CD-NSPCs in the contralateral hemisphere or within the tumor in addition to systemic 5-FC. The NSPCs migrated to the tumor across the corpus callosum, and treatment resulted in significantly reduced tumor size and improved animal survival.[86]

These initial studies of using NSPCs in the treatment of brain metastases are promising. NSPCs theoretically are advantageous due to tumor tropism and the flexibility in engineering these cells to deliver certain compounds or genes.[87] However, several questions must be answered before this therapy can be translated into patients with brain metastasis. Specifically, concerns of tumorigenic potential and immunogenicity of the NSPCs need to be studied to determine safety.

SUMMARY

This is an interesting period in neuro-oncology and the treatment of metastatic brain tumors. Emerging systemic chemotherapy allows for greater control and remission of primary lesions. Advanced neuroimaging techniques allow for greater visualization and characterization of metastases. Improved surgical techniques and technology allow for less invasive removal of metastases. SRS and WBRT are being used to improve local and distant controls, respectively. However, other techniques such as local sensitizers allow for more focused irradiation and subsequent decrease in harmful side effects. As more is learned about the genetic and genomic profiles of these tumors, molecular and stem cell–associated therapies will play larger roles in the treatment of brain metastases. It is clear that not all brain metastases behave the same, and individualized treatment will become the rule rather than the exception in this endeavor.

REFERENCES

1. Gavrilovic IT, Posner JB. Brain metastases: epidemiology and pathophysiology. J Neurooncol 2005; 75(1):5–14.
2. Shaffrey ME, Mut M, Asher AL, et al. Brain metastases. Curr Probl Surg 2004;41(8):665–741.
3. Jukich PJ, McCarthy BJ, Surawicz TS, et al. Trends in incidence of primary brain tumors in the United States, 1985–1994. Neuro Oncol 2001;3(3):141–51.
4. Kalkanis SN, Kondziolka D, Gaspar LE, et al. The role of surgical resection in the management of newly diagnosed brain metastases: a systematic review and evidence-based clinical practice guideline. J Neurooncol 2010;96(1):33–43.

5. Bindal AK, Bindal RK, Hess KR, et al. Surgery versus radiosurgery in the treatment of brain metastasis. J Neurosurg 1996;84(5):748–54.

6. Patchell RA, Tibbs PA, Regine WF, et al. Postoperative radiotherapy in the treatment of single metastases to the brain: a randomized trial. JAMA 1998; 280(17):1485–9.

7. Al-Shamy G, Sawaya R. Management of brain metastases: the indispensable role of surgery. J Neurooncol 2009;92(3):275–82.

8. Muacevic A, Wowra B, Siefert A, et al. Microsurgery plus whole brain irradiation versus Gamma Knife surgery alone for treatment of single metastases to the brain: a randomized controlled multicentre phase III trial. J Neurooncol 2008;87(3):299–307.

9. Gaspar LE, Mehta MP, Patchell RA, et al. The role of whole brain radiation therapy in the management of newly diagnosed brain metastases: a systematic review and evidence-based clinical practice guideline. J Neurooncol 2010;96(1):17–32.

10. Mehta MP, Paleologos NA, Mikkelsen T, et al. The role of chemotherapy in the management of newly diagnosed brain metastases: a systematic review and evidence-based clinical practice guideline. J Neurooncol 2010;96(1):71–83.

11. Linskey ME, Andrews DW, Asher AL, et al. The role of stereotactic radiosurgery in the management of patients with newly diagnosed brain metastases: a systematic review and evidence-based clinical practice guideline. J Neurooncol 2010;96(1):45–68.

12. Patchell RA, Tibbs PA, Walsh JW, et al. A randomized trial of surgery in the treatment of single metastases to the brain. N Engl J Med 1990;322(8):494–500.

13. Li B, Yu J, Suntharalingam M, et al. Comparison of three treatment options for single brain metastasis from lung cancer. Int J Cancer 2000;90(1):37–45.

14. Rades D, Pluemer A, Veninga T, et al. Whole-brain radiotherapy versus stereotactic radiosurgery for patients in recursive partitioning analysis classes 1 and 2 with 1 to 3 brain metastases. Cancer 2007; 110(10):2285–92.

15. Aoyama H, Shirato H, Tago M, et al. Stereotactic radiosurgery plus whole-brain radiation therapy vs stereotactic radiosurgery alone for treatment of brain metastases: a randomized controlled trial. JAMA 2006;295(21):2483–91.

16. Welzel G, Fleckenstein K, Schaefer J, et al. Memory function before and after whole brain radiotherapy in patients with and without brain metastases. Int J Radiat Oncol Biol Phys 2008;72(5):1311–8.

17. Chang EL, Wefel JS, Hess KR, et al. Neurocognition in patients with brain metastases treated with radiosurgery or radiosurgery plus whole-brain irradiation: a randomised controlled trial. Lancet Oncol 2009; 10(11):1037–44.

18. Arbit E, Wronski M, Burt M, et al. The treatment of patients with recurrent brain metastases. A retrospective analysis of 109 patients with nonsmall cell lung cancer. Cancer 1995;76(5):765–73.

19. Olson JJ, Paleologos NA, Gaspar LE, et al. The role of emerging and investigational therapies for metastatic brain tumors: a systematic review and evidence-based clinical practice guideline of selected topics. J Neurooncol 2010;96(1):115–42.

20. DeAngelis LM, Currie VE, Kim JH, et al. The combined use of radiation therapy and lonidamine in the treatment of brain metastases. J Neurooncol 1989;7(3):241–7.

21. Knisely JP, Berkey B, Chakravarti A, et al. A phase III study of conventional radiation therapy plus thalidomide versus conventional radiation therapy for multiple brain metastases (RTOG 0118). Int J Radiat Oncol Biol Phys 2008;71(1):79–86.

22. Woodburn KW. Intracellular localization of the radiation enhancer motexafin gadolinium using interferometric Fourier fluorescence microscopy. J Pharmacol Exp Ther 2001;297(3):888–94.

23. Evens AM, Balasubramanian L, Gordon LI. Motexafin gadolinium induces oxidative stress and apoptosis in hematologic malignancies. Curr Treat Options Oncol 2005;6(4):289–96.

24. Carde P, Timmerman R, Mehta MP, et al. Multicenter phase Ib/II trial of the radiation enhancer motexafin gadolinium in patients with brain metastases. J Clin Oncol 2001;19(7):2074–83.

25. Mehta MP, Rodrigus P, Terhaard CH, et al. Survival and neurologic outcomes in a randomized trial of motexafin gadolinium and whole-brain radiation therapy in brain metastases. J Clin Oncol 2003; 21(13):2529–36.

26. Mehta MP, Shapiro WR, Phan SC, et al. Motexafin gadolinium combined with prompt whole brain radiotherapy prolongs time to neurologic progression in non-small-cell lung cancer patients with brain metastases: results of a phase III trial. Int J Radiat Oncol Biol Phys 2009;73(4):1069–76.

27. Rockwell S, Kelley M. RSR13, a synthetic allosteric modifier of hemoglobin, as an adjunct to radiotherapy: preliminary studies with EMT6 cells and tumors and normal tissues in mice. Radiat Oncol Investig 1998;6(5):199–208.

28. Shaw E, Scott C, Suh J, et al. RSR13 plus cranial radiation therapy in patients with brain metastases: comparison with the Radiation Therapy Oncology Group Recursive Partitioning Analysis Brain Metastases Database. J Clin Oncol 2003;21(12):2364–71.

29. Stea B, Suh JH, Boyd AP, et al. Whole-brain radiotherapy with or without efaproxiral for the treatment of brain metastases: determinants of response and its prognostic value for subsequent survival. Int J Radiat Oncol Biol Phys 2006;64(4):1023–30.

30. Stock RG, Stone NN. Current topics in the treatment of prostate cancer with low-dose-rate brachytherapy. Urol Clin North Am 2010;37(1):83–96, table of contents.

31. Toita T. Current status and perspectives of brachytherapy for cervical cancer. Int J Clin Oncol 2009; 14(1):25–30.

32. Polgar C, Major T. Current status and perspectives of brachytherapy for breast cancer. Int J Clin Oncol 2009;14(1):7–24.

33. Alesch F, Hawliczek R, Koos WT. Interstitial irradiation of brain metastases. Acta Neurochir Suppl 1995;63:29–34.

34. Bernstein M, Cabantog A, Laperriere N, et al. Brachytherapy for recurrent single brain metastasis. Can J Neurol Sci 1995;22(1):13–6.

35. Rogers LR, Rock JP, Sills AK, et al. Results of a phase II trial of the GliaSite radiation therapy system for the treatment of newly diagnosed, resected single brain metastases. J Neurosurg 2006; 105(3):375–84.

36. Bogart JA, Ungureanu C, Shihadeh E, et al. Resection and permanent I-125 brachytherapy without whole brain irradiation for solitary brain metastasis from non-small cell lung carcinoma. J Neurooncol 1999;44(1):53–7.

37. Dagnew E, Kanski J, McDermott MW, et al. Management of newly diagnosed single brain metastasis using resection and permanent iodine-125 seeds without initial whole-brain radiotherapy: a two institution experience. Neurosurg Focus 2007;22(3):E3.

38. McGirt MJ, Than KD, Weingart JD, et al. Gliadel (BCNU) wafer plus concomitant temozolomide therapy after primary resection of glioblastoma multiforme. J Neurosurg 2009;110(3):583–8.

39. Ewend MG, Brem S, Gilbert M, et al. Treatment of single brain metastasis with resection, intracavity carmustine polymer wafers, and radiation therapy is safe and provides excellent local control. Clin Cancer Res 2007;13(12):3637–41.

40. Nakagawa H, Maeda N, Tsuzuki T, et al. Intracavitary chemotherapy with 5-fluoro-2′-deoxyuridine (FdUrd) in malignant brain tumors. Jpn J Clin Oncol 2001; 31(6):251–8.

41. Ewend MG, Sampath P, Williams JA, et al. Local delivery of chemotherapy prolongs survival in experimental brain metastases from breast carcinoma. Neurosurgery 1998;43(5):1185–93.

42. Eljamel MS. New light on the brain: the role of photosensitizing agents and laser light in the management of invasive intracranial tumors. Technol Cancer Res Treat 2003;2(4):303–9.

43. Aziz F, Telara S, Moseley H, et al. Photodynamic therapy adjuvant to surgery in metastatic carcinoma in brain. Photodiagnosis Photodyn Ther 2009; 6(3–4):227–30.

44. Curry WT Jr, Cosgrove GR, Hochberg FH, et al. Stereotactic interstitial radiosurgery for cerebral metastases. J Neurosurg 2005;103(4):630–5.

45. Pantazis G, Trippel M, Birg W, et al. Stereotactic interstitial radiosurgery with the Photon Radiosurgery System (PRS) for metastatic brain tumors: a prospective single-center clinical trial. Int J Radiat Oncol Biol Phys 2009;75(5):1392–400.

46. Fan M, Ascher PW, Schrottner O, et al. Interstitial 1.06 Nd:YAG laser thermotherapy for brain tumors under real-time monitoring of MRI: experimental study and phase I clinical trial. J Clin Laser Med Surg 1992;10(5):355–61.

47. Carpentier A, McNichols RJ, Stafford RJ, et al. Real-time magnetic resonance-guided laser thermal therapy for focal metastatic brain tumors. Neurosurgery 2008;63(1 Suppl 1):ONS21–8 [discussion: ONS28–9].

48. Schwartz JA, Shetty AM, Price RE, et al. Feasibility study of particle-assisted laser ablation of brain tumors in orthotopic canine model. Cancer Res 2009;69(4):1659–67.

49. Stupp R, Mason WP, van den Bent MJ, et al. Radiotherapy plus concomitant and adjuvant temozolomide for glioblastoma. N Engl J Med 2005;352(10): 987–96.

50. Hegi ME, Diserens AC, Gorlia T, et al. MGMT gene silencing and benefit from temozolomide in glioblastoma. N Engl J Med 2005;352(10):997–1003.

51. Reid JM, Stevens DC, Rubin J, et al. Pharmacokinetics of 3-methyl-(triazen-1-yl)imidazole-4-carboximide following administration of temozolomide to patients with advanced cancer. Clin Cancer Res 1997;3(12 Pt 1):2393–8.

52. Athanassiou H, Synodinou M, Maragoudakis E, et al. Randomized phase II study of temozolomide and radiotherapy compared with radiotherapy alone in newly diagnosed glioblastoma multiforme. J Clin Oncol 2005;23(10):2372–7.

53. Verger E, Gil M, Yaya R, et al. Temozolomide and concomitant whole brain radiotherapy in patients with brain metastases: a phase II randomized trial. Int J Radiat Oncol Biol Phys 2005;61(1):185–91.

54. Wu PF, Kuo KT, Kuo LT, et al. O(6)-Methylguanine-DNA methyltransferase expression and prognostic value in brain metastases of lung cancers. Lung Cancer 2010;68(3):484–90.

55. Ingold B, Schraml P, Heppner FL, et al. Homogeneous MGMT immunoreactivity correlates with an unmethylated MGMT promoter status in brain metastases of various solid tumors. PLoS One 2009;4(3):e4775.

56. Avril MF, Aamdal S, Grob JJ, et al. Fotemustine compared with dacarbazine in patients with disseminated malignant melanoma: a phase III study. J Clin Oncol 2004;22(6):1118–25.

57. Mornex F, Thomas L, Mohr P, et al. A prospective randomized multicentre phase III trial of fotemustine plus whole brain irradiation versus fotemustine alone in cerebral metastases of malignant melanoma. Melanoma Res 2003;13(1):97–103.

58. Yadav AK, Renfrow JJ, Scholtens DM, et al. Monosomy of chromosome 10 associated with dysregulation of epidermal growth factor signaling in glioblastomas. JAMA 2009;302(3):276–89.

59. Bredel M, Scholtens DM, Harsh GR, et al. A network model of a cooperative genetic landscape in brain tumors. JAMA 2009;302(3):261–75.

60. Matsumoto S, Takahashi K, Iwakawa R, et al. Frequent EGFR mutations in brain metastases of lung adenocarcinoma. Int J Cancer 2006;119(6):1491–4.

61. Shimato S, Mitsudomi T, Kosaka T, et al. EGFR mutations in patients with brain metastases from lung cancer: association with the efficacy of gefitinib. Neuro Oncol 2006;8(2):137–44.

62. Lynch TJ, Bell DW, Sordella R, et al. Activating mutations in the epidermal growth factor receptor underlying responsiveness of non-small-cell lung cancer to gefitinib. N Engl J Med 2004;350(21):2129–39.

63. Yano S, Shinohara H, Herbst RS, et al. Expression of vascular endothelial growth factor is necessary but not sufficient for production and growth of brain metastasis. Cancer Res 2000;60(17):4959–67.

64. Labidi SI, Bachelot T, Ray-Coquard I, et al. Bevacizumab and paclitaxel for breast cancer patients with central nervous system metastases: a case series. Clin Breast Cancer 2009;9(2):118–21.

65. De Braganca KC, Janjigian YY, Azzoli CG, et al. Efficacy and safety of bevacizumab in active brain metastases from non-small cell lung cancer. J Neurooncol 2010. [Epub ahead of print].

66. Gordon MS, Margolin K, Talpaz M, et al. Phase I safety and pharmacokinetic study of recombinant human anti-vascular endothelial growth factor in patients with advanced cancer. J Clin Oncol 2001; 19(3):843–50.

67. Besse B, Lasserre SF, Compton P, et al. Bevacizumab safety in patients with central nervous system metastases. Clin Cancer Res 2010;16(1):269–78.

68. Bos PD, Zhang XH, Nadal C, et al. Genes that mediate breast cancer metastasis to the brain. Nature 2009;459(7249):1005–9.

69. Pommier SJ, Quan GG, Christante D, et al. Characterizing the HER2/neu status and metastatic potential of breast cancer stem/progenitor cells. Ann Surg Oncol 2010;17(2):613–23.

70. Klein A, Olendrowitz C, Schmutzler R, et al. Identification of brain- and bone-specific breast cancer metastasis genes. Cancer Lett 2009;276(2):212–20.

71. Grinberg-Rashi H, Ofek E, Perelman M, et al. The expression of three genes in primary non-small cell lung cancer is associated with metastatic spread to the brain. Clin Cancer Res 2009;15(5):1755–61.

72. Hamilton A. The division of the differentiated cells in the central nervous system of the white rate. J Comp Neurol 1901;11:297–320.

73. Kershman J. The medulloblast and the medulloblastoma. Arch Neurol Psychiatry 1938;40:937–67.

74. Bryans WA. Mitotic activity in the brain of the adult white rat. Anat Rec 1959;133:65–71.

75. Altman J. Proliferation and migration of undifferentiated precursor cells in the rat during postnatal gliogenesis. Exp Neurol 1966;16(3):263–78.

76. Altman J, Das GD. Autoradiographic and histological evidence of postnatal hippocampal neurogenesis in rats. J Comp Neurol 1965;124(3): 319–35.

77. Dacey ML, Wallace RB. Postnatal neurogenesis in the feline cerebellum: a structural-functional investigation. Acta Neurobiol Exp (Wars) 1974;34(2):253–63.

78. Kaplan MS, Hinds JW. Neurogenesis in the adult rat: electron microscopic analysis of light radioautographs. Science 1977;197(4308):1092–4.

79. Messier B, Leblond CP, Smart I. Presence of DNA synthesis and mitosis in the brain of young adult mice. Exp Cell Res 1958;14(1):224–6.

80. Paton JA, Nottebohm FN. Neurons generated in the adult brain are recruited into functional circuits. Science 1984;225(4666):1046–8.

81. Goldman SA, Nottebohm F. Neuronal production, migration, and differentiation in a vocal control nucleus of the adult female canary brain. Proc Natl Acad Sci U S A 1983;80(8):2390–4.

82. Reynolds BA, Weiss S. Generation of neurons and astrocytes from isolated cells of the adult mammalian central nervous system. Science 1992; 255(5052):1707–10.

83. Aboody KS, Brown A, Rainov NG, et al. Neural stem cells display extensive tropism for pathology in adult brain: evidence from intracranial gliomas. Proc Natl Acad Sci U S A 2000;97(23):12846–51.

84. Schmidt NO, Przylecki W, Yang W, et al. Brain tumor tropism of transplanted human neural stem cells is induced by vascular endothelial growth factor. Neoplasia 2005;7(6):623–9.

85. Aboody KS, Najbauer J, Schmidt NO, et al. Targeting of melanoma brain metastases using engineered neural stem/progenitor cells. Neuro Oncol 2006;8(2): 119–26.

86. Joo KM, Park IH, Shin JY, et al. Human neural stem cells can target and deliver therapeutic genes to breast cancer brain metastases. Mol Ther 2009; 17(3):570–5.

87. Aboody KS, Najbauer J, Danks MK. Stem and progenitor cell-mediated tumor selective gene therapy. Gene Ther 2008;15(10):739–52.

Evidence-Based Guidelines for the Management of Brain Metastases

Sandeep S. Bhangoo, MS, MD[a], Mark E. Linskey, MD[b,c],
Steven N. Kalkanis, MD[a,*]

KEYWORDS
- Brain metastases • Surgical resection • Radiotherapy
- Stereotactic radiosurgery • Chemotherapy
- Systemic review • Practice guidelines

Metastatic tumors of the brain are defined as secondary lesions that have spread from a primary cancer originating in another system. It is difficult to generate precise data on the incidence of these lesions because they are poorly studied. It is estimated that 1.4 million Americans are diagnosed with cancer every year. Approximately 20% to 40% of these patients with systemic cancer will develop a metastasis to the brain making this disease roughly 4 to 5 times more common than primary brain tumors.[1]

Any attempt to develop strong guidelines based on evidence requires careful definition of the target population, the interventions used, and the measured outcomes. The concept of defining a disease as a metastatic lesion originating from elsewhere implies a wide variation in pathologic presentation and natural course that can depend on several factors. A summary of these variables can be categorized into patient-specific (age, neurologic status, and presence of medical co-morbidities), brain lesion-specific (size, location, and number of brain lesions), and tumor-specific (extent and prognosis of the systemic cancer). These 8 variables alone can vary widely from patient to patient, making a rigid algorithm for patient treatment almost impossible to devise given the current state of medical knowledge. Nevertheless, a systematic review of the large number of peer-reviewed publications on this subject can be extremely useful to the practitioners of neurosurgery, radiation oncology, neuro-oncology, and also medical oncology.

The American Association of Neurologic Surgeons (AANS), the Congress of Neurologic Surgeons (CNS), and the AANS/CNS Joint Tumor Section jointly funded an initiative to set up a Management of Brain Metastases Guidelne (MBMG) panel to address this issue.[2] The panel included 17 clinical experts from surgical neuro-oncology, radiation oncology, and medical neuro-oncology. A comprehensive electronic literature search from the past 20 years was initiated with articles dating as recently as April 2009. The search yielded 16,966 candidate articles that were subsequently screened for relevance to the particular topic. Screened articles were then reviewed in accordance to the evidence classification adopted by the AANS/CNS (**Table 1**). Each eligible study was assigned to a class based on study design

The authors have nothing to disclose.

[a] Department of Neurosurgery, Henry Ford Health System, Hermelin Brain Tumor Center, 2799 West Grand Boulevard, K-11, Detroit, MI 48202, USA

[b] Department of Neurosurgery, University of California-Irvine Medical Center, 101 The City Drive South Building 56, Suite 400, Orange, CA 92868, USA

[c] Department of Neurological Surgery, University of California-Irvine Medical Center, 101 The City Drive South, Building 56, Suite 400, Orange, CA 92868, USA

* Corresponding author.

E-mail address: skalkan1@hfhs.org

Neurosurg Clin N Am 22 (2011) 97–104
doi:10.1016/j.nec.2010.09.001
1042-3680/11/$ — see front matter © 2011 Elsevier Inc. All rights reserved.

alone. The levels of recommendations made (see **Table 1**) were based on aspects of study quality as well as design. If there was a consensus by the panel regarding methodological concerns of certain studies, for example, it would warrant a decrease in the level of recommendation.

The panel organized its review around 8 clinical questions that corresponded to the 8 practice guideline papers[3–10] that form the major subject of this article. The 8 questions were segregated by target population into 3 categories: 4 questions pertained to patients with newly diagnosed brain metastasis, 1 question pertained to previously treated patients who present with recurrent or progressive metastasis, and 3 questions pertained to all patients with brain metastasis.

It is thought that patients with untreated brain metastasis have a median survival of approximately 1 month with mortality usually related to neurologic compromise.[11] The ultimate goal of treatment is to minimize the effects of these lesions while preserving neurologic function. This goal acknowledges the limitations in attempting to prolong overall survival by altering the course of systemic disease outside the nervous system. There are 3 main treatments that are considered for patients presenting with a newly diagnosed brain metastasis: whole brain radiation therapy, surgical resection, and stereotactic radiosurgery. Each is thought to provide benefit in certain clinical scenarios and is the primary focus of the review.

THE ROLE OF RADIATION

Whole-brain radiation therapy (WBRT) has been the standard treatment for all patients with brain metastasis. The rationale behind treatment outside of the tumor bed is the prevention of widely disseminated recurrent metastases throughout the brain. Because the brain can generally tolerate radiation better than other organs, WBRT also has a role in local tumor control. There are certain histopathologic tumor subgroups (small cell lung cancer, leukemia, lymphoma, germ cell tumors, multiple myeloma) that are considered radiosensitive and treated almost exclusively with WBRT. Conversely, other tumor histopathologies, such as melanoma, renal cell carcinoma, and sarcoma, are radioresistant. Between these extremes lay the vast majority of patients with common tumor histopathologies, such as breast cancer and non-small-cell lung cancer. Given the wide variety of presentations based on the variables previously mentioned, a general guideline cannot be applied to everyone. Rather, it is recommended that the guidelines be taken in the context of a multidisciplinary treatment paradigm to choose the optimal course of therapy. A risk to consider when giving WBRT is the development of neurocognitive deficits. These deficits can be subtle and easily missed on many routine medical examinations or basic mental evaluations, such as the Mini-Mental Status Examination. Nevertheless, they can be disturbing to both patients and families.

WBRT Alone versus Combination Surgical Resection and WBRT

Seven studies were reviewed by the MBMG panel to generate a Level 1 recommendation stating that

Table 1
AANS/CNS evidence classes and levels of recommendation

Evidence Classification	
Class I	Evidence provided by 1 or more well-designed randomized controlled clinical trials, including overview (meta-analyses) of such trials
Class II	Evidence provided by well-designed observational studies with concurrent controls (eg, case control and cohort studies)
Class III	Evidence provided by expert opinion, case series, case reports, and studies with historical controls
Levels of Recommendation	
Level 1	Generally accepted principles for patient management that reflect a high degree of clinical certainty (usually this requires Class I evidence, which directly addresses the clinical questions or overwhelming Class II evidence when circumstances preclude randomized clinical trials)
Level 2	Recommendations for patient management that reflect clinical certainty (usually this requires Class II evidence or a strong consensus of Class III evidence)
Level 3	Other strategies for patient management for which the clinical utility is uncertain (inconclusive or conflicting evidence or opinion)

Class I evidence supports the combination of surgical resection plus postoperative WBRT, as compared with WBRT alone, in patients with good performance status (functionally independent and spending less than 50% of the time in bed) and limited extracranial disease.[9] There is insufficient evidence to make a recommendation for patients with poor performance scores, advanced systemic disease, or multiple brain metastases.

Optimal Dosing/Fractionation Schedule for WBRT

A total of 23 studies were reviewed by the MBMG panel to generate a Level 1 recommendation stating that Class I evidence suggests that altered dose/fractionation schedules of WBRT do not result in significant differences in median survival, local control, or neurocognitive outcomes when compared with standard WBRT dose/fractionation. (ie, 30 Gy in 10 fractions or a biologically effective dose [BED] of 39 Gy_{10}). This evidence was generated by performing a meta-analysis of the multiple studies by expressing several different radiation schedules in terms of the BED, which takes into account the total dose of radiation, fraction size, and overall time to deliver the radiation and presume repair of irradiated tissue. The standard dose previously mentioned served as the control dose; none of the trials with low-dose regimens or high-dose regimens relative to the control dose showed a significant difference in overall survival.

WBRT in Different Tumor Histopathologies

The MBMG panel was able to identify only 1 Class III article on this subject and was, therefore, unable to support the choice of any particular dose/fractionation regimen based on histopathology.

THE ROLE OF SURGERY

The question of surgical resection arises in patients presenting with brain metastasis. It is the responsibility of the treating neurosurgeon to determine whether it is possible to resect the lesion without causing further neurologic deficit. The brain lesion-specific variables previously mentioned are critically important factors when considering options other than radiation alone. The brain-lesion specific variables of size, number, and location of lesions can be best determined by a gadolinium-enhanced MRI scan or, if unavailable, CT scan with contrast of the brain.

For *size*, surgical resection can be thought of as a cytoreductive strategy to reduce the overall tumor burden for other therapies. In this scenario, tumors less than 0.5 cm in diameter may be too small to warrant an exclusive surgical intervention; whereas, those greater than 3 cm may not be effectively treated by any modality other than surgery. Size may be a complicating factor if there is sufficient mass effect to compromise neurologic function. An easily accessible tumor in the posterior fossa or temporal lobe, for example, can cause significant neurologic compromise because of the risk of compression to adjacent structures. In these scenarios, there may not be sufficient time for nonsurgical therapies to work.

For *number*, it is generally thought that resection of more than 1 lesion via multiple craniotomies is inadvisable. One may consider surgery for multiple, large metastatic lesions with mass effect that may be amenable to surgery or multiple lesions that may be accessible through a single craniotomy. Another indication for surgery in the face of multiple metastases is for biopsy for diagnosis in the absence of a known primary source. Approximately 37% to 50% of patients with brain metastases with primary cancers that are solid tumors will present with only 1 lesion.[1,12,13] Given this statistic, many patients will be candidates for surgical resection.

Regarding *location*, the question arises as to whether the lesion is accessible through standard neurosurgical approaches with minimal risk of damage to eloquent structures. Again the extremes of a 1-cm lesion in the superficial cortex of the right frontal lobe (resectable) versus in the midbrain (nonresectable) bound a variety of scenarios that should be evaluated on a case by case basis by the treating neurosurgeon.

Combination Surgical Resection Plus WBRT versus Surgical Resection Alone

The MBMG panel reviewed 4 studies, including 1 randomized control trial (RCT). Based on these studies, a Level 1 recommendation stated that combination surgical resection followed by WBRT represents a superior treatment modality, in terms of improving tumor control at the original site of the metastasis and in the brain overall, when compared with surgical resection alone.[5] These patients may still benefit from aggressive local control even with uncontrolled systemic disease. However, they usually have a Karnofsky Performance Score (KPS) greater than or equal to 70. The outcomes of overall survival and time with KPS greater than or equal to 70 were not significantly different. This finding may be caused by progression of systemic disease.

THE ROLE OF STEREOTACTIC RADIOSURGERY

Stereotactic radiosurgery (SRS) delivers multiple radiation beams to a specified target volume, thereby delivering a much higher dose compared with the surrounding tissue. It has been used in functional and vascular neurosurgical pathologies as well as neuro-oncology. SRS is a noninvasive modality that can safely target tumor volumes less than 10 mL. Because most metastatic lesions are spherical, this volume approximates to a lesion that is 3 cm in diameter. In addition, the evidence recommendations for SRS do not apply to lesions causing greater than 1cm of midline shift from mass effect. Although SRS has been seen as an alternative to surgery and WBRT, it may also be used in combination treatments. Given the number of variations to this modality, the MBMG panel made several recommendations.

WBRT versus Combination SRS and WBRT

Five studies were reviewed by the MBMG panel. The evidence reviewed generated a total of 4 recommendations that consistently showed the superiority of SRS combined with WBRT compared with WBRT alone, but differed by strength of recommendation as well as by inclusion criteria and outcomes.[6] The first Level 1 recommendation for combination SRS plus WBRT was for patients with single metastases with a KPS greater than or equal to 70, a group which demonstrated significantly longer patient survival compared with patients treated with WBRT alone. The second Level 1 recommendation for combination SRS and WBRT was for patients with 1 to 4 metastatic lesions with a KPS greater than or equal to 70, a group which had better local tumor control and maintenance of functional status compared with WBRT alone. For the outcome of significantly longer patient survival, a Level 2 recommendation stated that the combination of SRS and WBRT is superior in patients with 2 to 3 metastatic lesions. Finally, a Level 3 recommendation stated that there is Class III evidence demonstrating that single-dose SRS along with WBRT is superior to WBRT alone for improving patient survival for patients with single or multiple brain metastases and a KPS less than 70.

Combination SRS and WBRT versus SRS Alone

Given the strong evidence in favor of SRS and WBRT when compared with WBRT alone, the next logical question was to explore what evidence supports the opposite approach. SRS alone may be an advantage to patients in that one therapy session is required. The entire brain is not exposed to radiation in SRS; furthermore, there is a risk of potential neurocognitive deficits with the use of WBRT, although this has not been well studied because the effects may be subtle and variable. The risk, however, is the loss of control of distant tumor recurrence that is thought to be minimized by WBRT. Although it may be tempting to consider SRS as a substitute for surgery, one cannot ignore the fact that it may have biologic effects similar to WBRT. Eleven studies were reviewed by the MBMG panel that generated a Level 2 recommendation stating that SRS alone may provide an equivalent survival advantage for patients with brain metastases compared with combined WBRT and SRS. There is conflicting Class I and II evidence regarding the risk of both local and distant recurrence when SRS is used in isolation and Class I evidence demonstrates a lower risk of distant recurrence with WBRT. Therefore, regular careful surveillance is warranted for patients treated with SRS alone to provide early identification of local and distant recurrences so that salvage therapy can be initiated at the soonest possible time.

SRS Alone versus WBRT Alone

Four Class II studies were reviewed that consistently showed that SRS alone yielded a significant survival advantage when compared with WBRT alone. However, because the supporting data was weak, the MBMG panel generated a Level 3 recommendation stating that single-dose SRS alone appears to be superior to WBRT alone for patients with up to 3 metastatic brain tumors in terms of a patient survival advantage.

Combination Surgery and WBRT versus SRS Alone

The MBMG panel recognized the importance of this comparison. Four studies were found but 1 was noted to be underpowered because it was closed prematurely and the Class II data generated conflicting results. A Level 3 recommendation stated that this evidence suggests that SRS alone may provide equivalent functional and survival outcomes compared with the combination of surgery and WBRT for patients with single brain metastases, so long as ready detection of distant site failure and salvage SRS are possible.

Combination Surgical Resection and WBRT versus Combination SRS and WBRT

The guidelines presented so far clearly show a significant benefit to combination therapies when compared with individual ones. Given this information, the question arises as to which combination is superior. In the case of the combination surgical resection and WBRT, versus combinations SRS and WBRT, the MBMG panel identified only 4 retrospective studies on this comparison. The panel issued a Level 2 recommendation stating that both combinations represent effective treatment strategies, resulting in equal survival rates.

The SRS recommendations were based on a single-dose application of SRS. The panel intended to study the role of multidose SRS but the studies found were insufficient to generate recommendations. The situation was also similar for the role of local radiotherapy. Finally, the therapy of surgical resection combined with postoperative SRS to the tumor bed was another topic that did not have enough studies to warrant a review.

THE ROLE OF CHEMOTHERAPY

Although chemotherapy is a standard mode of treatment in many systemic cancers, its use in the brain has been traditionally more limited. The blood-brain barrier (BBB) limits the penetration of most substances into the brain parenchyma. Although there is some breakdown of the BBB around metastatic lesions, it is thought that drug concentrations within these lesions are still limited secondary to active efflux mechanisms.

The guideline panel was interested in the following treatment paradigms[3]:

- WBRT versus WBRT plus chemotherapy
- Chemotherapy versus chemotherapy plus WBRT
- Concurrent WBRT and chemotherapy versus chemotherapy and delayed WBRT
- Chemotherapy first, then WBRT versus WBRT first, then chemotherapy.

The panel concluded that there is no clear survival benefit seen from the addition of chemotherapy to any WBRT paradigm. Therefore, a Level 1 recommendation was made against the routine use of chemotherapy in patients with a newly diagnosed brain metastasis.[3]

There are several points to make regarding this recommendation. First, a complicating factor for any general recommendation on chemotherapy usage in metastasis is that such a recommendation would overlook the variability of different tumor histologies and chemotherapeutic agents as well as the unique interactions that may occur with every possible combination. The panel noted, for example, that metastatic germinomas are chemosensitive and should not fall under this recommendation. Most of the studies reviewed here were

limited to non-small cell lung cancer and breast cancer. Second, the panel was unable to find studies that distinguished between chemotherapy naïve patients and those who had prior treatment for their systemic disease. Third, the studies reviewed did not have the same primary endpoint of overall survival. Finally, the panel recommended further enrollment in chemotherapy-based trials.[3]

RECURRENT OR PROGRESSIVE BRAIN METASTASIS

Given the difficulties in variability previously discussed with patients who present with newly diagnosed brain metastasis, one can expect an even greater number of variables to consider when patients develop recurrent metastasis or have progression of growth despite the first line of treatment. For patients who survive long enough to experience this scenario, there is no consensus on how to proceed with therapy.

The MBMG panel first addressed the evidence regarding the use of any of the previously discussed therapies (ie, WBRT, surgery, SRS, or chemotherapy).[10] On this issue, 30 studies were reviewed but no Class I or II studies were found. A Level 3 recommendation stated that treatment should be individualized based on the following factors: neurologic functional status, extent of systemic disease, volume and number of metastases, recurrence or progression at the original tumor site versus a new site, and previous treatments and histopathology of the tumor. Enrollment in clinical trials is encouraged. Considering these factors, the following options can be considered: no further treatment (supportive care), reirradiation (SRS or WBRT), surgical excision, or to a lesser extent, chemotherapy.

Finally, although the MBMG panel wished to examine the impact of differing tumor histopathologies on outcomes in patients with recurrence or progression treated with WBRT, no studies were found to be able to issue any recommendations.

THE ROLE OF ANTICONVULSANTS

Like any mass lesion, brain metastases have been known to cause epileptic seizures. Because of this, many practitioners have been known to routinely start anticonvulsant medications upon diagnosis of these lesions regardless of whether patients have suffered a seizure. As these medications have significant side effects, there is a question of whether the risk of anticonvulsant usage outweighs the potential benefit of seizure prevention. Metastatic brain lesions are thought to possibly have different epileptogenic characteristics when compared with primary brain tumors, which usually infiltrate brain parenchyma unlike the more circumscribed metastatic tumors.

The review targeted the single question: Do prophylactic anticonvulsants decrease the risk of seizures in patients with metastatic brain lesions who have not had any seizures? The systematic review of this topic found a paucity of eligible studies, with none showing a benefit for prophylactic therapy.[4] Therefore, the Level 3 recommendation was that routine anticonvulsant use should not be recommended.[4]

THE ROLE OF STEROIDS

Corticosteroid therapy has been widely used in brain metastasis treatment. There are typically 3 scenarios in which steroids may be considered for administration. The first is upon initial or recurrent diagnosis, which usually comes about from patients presenting with neurologic symptoms. The second scenario is during the perioperative period for microsurgical or stereotactic radiosurgery to minimize symptoms related to the intervention. The final scenario is during the long-term course of WBRT. In typical patients, these scenarios are likely to overlap in time.

Steroids are thought to reduce edema through their glucocorticoid effect by downregulating proinflammatory transcription factors at the nuclear level; these effects are not instantaneous. There are known risks to chronic steroid use. In addition to the well-known side effects, such as Cushing's syndrome, myopathy, and psychosis, special consideration should be made of the combination of hyperglycemia and immunosuppression in increasing the risk of infection, especially perioperatively. As edema is thought to be the primary pathology that is treatable by steroids, it is also important to recognize the causal link between edema and its associated symptoms along with the capabilities of the steroids to work effectively on an individual basis before judging the success or failure of steroid therapy. For example, the use of steroids to reduce mass effect from a large cerebellar metastasis compressing the fourth ventricle and causing hydrocephalus may not sufficiently reduce the edema before patients undergo herniation. Similarly, consider the idea of steroid use alone on a temporal lobe metastasis in patients presenting with status epilepticus. In both cases, mass effect or peritumoral edema may be the causal agent, but selecting steroids as an exclusive therapy to reduce the neurologic symptoms will likely result in unfavorable outcomes.

Three general concepts were addressed in the review[8]: whether to administer steroids, what dose and kind of steroid to give, and how long the steroid should be administered. The outcome under question was not overall survival, but rather clinical neurologic symptom improvement.

For the question of whether to administer steroids, the target population was stratified according to symptoms relating to mass effect from edema. For clinically asymptomatic patients that demonstrate no mass effect on radiographic studies, there is insufficient evidence to make any recommendation. If patients are experiencing symptoms from mass effect, however, the panel's Level 3 recommendation is that corticosteroids can provide temporary symptomatic relief of symptoms related to increased intracranial pressure. For mild to moderate symptoms, the recommended dosage is 4 to 8 mg/day; whereas, more severe symptoms may have dosages increased up to 16 mg/day.

The panel made a Level 3 recommendation of dexamethasone as the steroid of choice for its low mineralocorticoid effects. As to the duration of therapy, the panel stated that individual factors, such as the severity of symptoms, coupled with an understanding of the consequences of the long-term sequelae should be considered before deciding the length of therapy. However, the panel made a Level 3 recommendation to taper the steroids, once started, over a 2-week period.

Given that steroid therapy alone has little effect on overall survival, the question that requires systematic analysis is whether the benefits of temporary steroid usage outweigh its risks. As the level of evidence is currently Class 3 at best, there is opportunity for addressing the questions of treatment dosages and durations because the panel was unable to identify any ongoing studies on these issues. Another potential avenue for investigation is the role of steroid therapy for symptomatic palliation during SRS, WBRT, or surgical treatment regimens.

THE ROLE OF EMERGING THERAPIES

Given the preponderance of new therapies under investigation, patients and their families will likely question treating physicians regarding these novel treatments that are usually not available outside clinical trials. It is difficult to systematically exhaust all these therapies in an evidence-based review. Nevertheless, the panel did attempt to address some of the emerging and investigational therapies that have been evaluated in clinical trials.[7]

Radiation Sensitizers

These agents are thought to increase the effectiveness of WBRT. The 2 agents reviewed were motexafin-gadolinium (MGd) and efaproxiral

(RSR 13) from data in 5 unique studies. The panel noted that a subgroup of subjects with non-small cell lung cancer who had received MGd early in an RCT had a prolongation of the time to neurologic progression; however, this was not borne out in the overall study population. Therefore, a Level 2 recommendation was made stating that currently these agents have not yet shown sufficient evidence to warrant their use.

Interstitial Therapies

The potential benefit of interstitial therapies is the ability to achieve local control without systemic dissemination of cytotoxic chemotherapy or radiation. However, there is a known risk of toxicity from these treatments. The panel reviewed 11 studies but was unable to generate any Level 1 or 2 recommendations. Currently, there is no evidence to support the use of interstitial modalities outside of clinical trials.

New Chemotherapeutic Agents

The panel reviewed 31 studies regarding the use of novel chemotherapeutic agents. The majority of these were on the subject of temozolomide (TMZ), which is widely used in the treatment of primary brain cancers. The panel issued a Level 2 recommendation stating that the addition of TMZ to WBRT in the treatment of melanoma metastasis is reasonable. Also, a Level 3 recommendation stated that there may be individual circumstances, based on multiple reports, where TMZ or fotemustine can benefit patients. Further investigations are warranted.

Molecular Targeted Agents

Molecular targeted agents have been incorporated into many cancer treatment paradigms in the last decade. There has been considerable progress in laboratory-based development and use of these agents, yet bedside application has lagged. The panel noted 2 molecular pathways that have received considerable attention: the epidermal growth factor and angiogenesis pathways. Six studies were found on the use of gefitinib, which blocks the epidermal growth factor receptor. From these studies, a Level 3 recommendation was made in the use of this agent in the treatment of brain metastases from non-small cell lung cancer. The angiogenesis pathway can be targeted by thalidomide and bevacizumab. No studies were found by the panel investigating their use in brain metastasis.

SUMMARY

Table 2 provides a summary of the number of articles reviewed by topic as well as the number of recommendations made in each section by level of evidence.[3-10] Although there were several overlaps within the review, the key recommendations are that for patients with newly diagnosed metastatic brain lesions, there is strong evidence for the involvement of radiation therapy, surgical therapy, and stereotactic radiosurgery in combination. There does not appear to be an established role for any chemotherapeutic agents at this time. For patients with recurrent or progressive brain metastases, individualization of therapies may be the best approach based on several variables discussed in this article. For all patients with brain metastasis, anticonvulsants can be held in

---

Table 2
Numerical summary of articles and recommendations by topic

Section Topic	Articles Reviewed	Eligible Studies	Level 1 Recommendations	Level 2 Recommendations	Level 3 Recommendations
Radiation therapy[a]	65	31	3	0	0
Surgical resection[a]	33	15	2	1	1
Stereotactic radiosurgery[a]	56	32	2	3	3
Chemotherapy	30	10	1	0	0
Retreatment	81	30	0	0	1
Anticonvulsant use	4	1	0	0	1
Steroid use	2	2	0	0	4
Novel therapies	125	59	0	2	2
Total	396	180	8	6	12

[a] There is some overlap in the articles reviewed and recommendations in these topics.

patients who have not suffered seizures, steroid use may be tailored to the patient's symptoms though they are not generally considered chemotherapy, and novel therapies currently under clinical investigation cannot yet be integrated into evidence-based guidelines as their efficacy remains unproven. Combination therapies spread across multiple medical disciplines; it becomes clear that single-specialty management of this disease is no longer sufficient to achieve quality care. Finally, there remain several questions to be resolved with evidence-based guidelines. The MBMG panel has indicated the need to review and update the guidelines every 5 years. Included in the panel's review were the names of trials currently underway that will likely make major contributions to future guidelines.

REFERENCES

1. Gavrilovic IT, Posner JB. Brain metastases: epidemiology and pathophysiology. J Neurooncol 2005; 75(1):5–14.
2. Kalkanis SN, Linskey ME. Evidence-based clinical practice parameter guidelines for the treatment of patients with metastatic brain tumors: introduction. J Neurooncol 2010;96(1):7–10.
3. Mehta MP, Paleologos NA, Mikkelsen T, et al. The role of chemotherapy in the management of newly diagnosed brain metastases: a systematic review and evidence-based clinical practice guideline. J Neurooncol 2010;96(1):71–83.
4. Mikkelsen T, Paleologos NA, Robinson PD, et al. The role of prophylactic anticonvulsants in the management of brain metastases: a systematic review and evidence-based clinical practice guideline. J Neurooncol 2010;96(1):97–102.
5. Kalkanis SN, Kondziolka D, Gaspar LE, et al. The role of surgical resection in the management of newly diagnosed brain metastases: a systematic review and evidence-based clinical practice guideline. J Neurooncol 2010;96(1):33–43.
6. Linskey ME, Andrews DW, Asher AL, et al. The role of stereotactic radiosurgery in the management of patients with newly diagnosed brain metastases: a systematic review and evidence-based clinical practice guideline. J Neurooncol 2010;96(1):45–68.
7. Olson JJ, Paleologos NA, Gaspar LE, et al. The role of emerging and investigational therapies for metastatic brain tumors: a systematic review and evidence-based clinical practice guideline of selected topics. J Neurooncol 2010;96(1):115–42.
8. Ryken TC, McDermott M, Robinson PD, et al. The role of steroids in the management of brain metastases: a systematic review and evidence-based clinical practice guideline. J Neurooncol 2010;96(1): 103–14.
9. Gaspar LE, Mehta MP, Patchell RA, et al. The role of whole brain radiation therapy in the management of newly diagnosed brain metastases: a systematic review and evidence-based clinical practice guideline. J Neurooncol 2010;96(1):17–32.
10. Ammirati M, Cobbs CS, Linskey ME, et al. The role of retreatment in the management of recurrent/progressive brain metastases: a systematic review and evidence-based clinical practice guideline. J Neurooncol 2010;96(1):85–96.
11. Patchell RA. The management of brain metastases. Cancer Treat Rev 2003;29(6):533–40.
12. Delattre JY, Krol G, Thaler HT, et al. Distribution of brain metastases. Arch Neurol 1988;45(7):741–4.
13. Deutsch M, Parsons JA, Mercado R. Radiotherapy for intracranial metastases. Cancer 1974;34(5): 1607–11.

Index

Note: Page numbers of article titles are in **boldface** type.

Neurosurg Clin N Am 22 (2011) 105–109
doi:10.1016/S1042-3680(10)00107-5
1042-3680/11/$ – see front matter © 2011 Elsevier Inc. All rights reserved.

Moving?

Make sure your subscription moves with you!

To notify us of your new address, find your **Clinics Account Number** (located on your mailing label above your name), and contact customer service at:

Email: journalscustomerservice-usa@elsevier.com

800-654-2452 (subscribers in the U.S. & Canada)
314-447-8871 (subscribers outside of the U.S. & Canada)

Fax number: 314-447-8029

Elsevier Health Sciences Division
Subscription Customer Service
3251 Riverport Lane
Maryland Heights, MO 63043

*To ensure uninterrupted delivery of your subscription, please notify us at least 4 weeks in advance of move.

Printed and bound by CPI Group (UK) Ltd, Croydon, CR0 4YY

03/10/2024

01040354-0003